Critical and Applied Approaches in Sexuality, Gender and Identity

Series Editor
Christina Richards
Calver, Derbyshire, UK

This series brings together scholars from a range of disciplines who have produced work which both informs the academy and, crucially, has real-world applied implications for a variety of different professions, including psychologists; psychiatrists; psychotherapists; counsellors; medical doctors; nurses; social workers; researchers and lecturers; governmental policy advisors; non-governmental policy advisors; and peer support workers, among others. The series critically considers intersections between sexuality and gender; practice and identity; and theoretical and applied arenas – as well as questioning, where appropriate, the nature or reality of the boundaries between them.

In short, it aims to build castles in the sky we can live in – after all the view is nothing, without a place to stand.

Editorial Board:
Christina Richards, Nottinghamshire Healthcare NHS Foundation Trust, UK
Jon Arcelus, Nottinghamshire Healthcare NHS Foundation Trust, UK
Surya Monro, University of Huddersfield, UK
Simon DuPlock, Metanoia Instutite, UK
Timo Nieder, Interdisciplinary Transgender Health Care Center Hamburg, Germany

More information about this series at
http://www.palgrave.com/gp/series/15443

Damien W. Riggs

Working with Transgender Young People and their Families

A Critical Developmental Approach

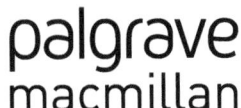

Damien W. Riggs
College of Education, Psychology and Social Work
Flinders University
Adelaide, SA, Australia

Critical and Applied Approaches in Sexuality, Gender and Identity
ISBN 978-3-030-14230-8   ISBN 978-3-030-14231-5 (Ebook)
https://doi.org/10.1007/978-3-030-14231-5

Library of Congress Control Number: 2019934466

© The Editor(s) (if applicable) and The Author(s), under exclusive licence to Springer Nature Switzerland AG 2019
This work is subject to copyright. All rights are solely and exclusively licensed by the Publisher, whether the whole or part of the material is concerned, specifically the rights of translation, reprinting, reuse of illustrations, recitation, broadcasting, reproduction on microfilms or in any other physical way, and transmission or information storage and retrieval, electronic adaptation, computer software, or by similar or dissimilar methodology now known or hereafter developed.
The use of general descriptive names, registered names, trademarks, service marks, etc. in this publication does not imply, even in the absence of a specific statement, that such names are exempt from the relevant protective laws and regulations and therefore free for general use.
The publisher, the authors and the editors are safe to assume that the advice and information in this book are believed to be true and accurate at the date of publication. Neither the publisher nor the authors or the editors give a warranty, express or implied, with respect to the material contained herein or for any errors or omissions that may have been made. The publisher remains neutral with regard to jurisdictional claims in published maps and institutional affiliations.

Cover illustration: ©Lilith Saintclaire

This Palgrave Macmillan imprint is published by the registered company Springer Nature Switzerland AG.
The registered company address is: Gewerbestrasse 11, 6330 Cham, Switzerland

For two special people, who lead me to this path

Preface

My intentions for this book started from a very simple premise: transgender young people exist, they know who they are, and they deserve all of the support and care we can give them. From the first transgender young person I worked with over a decade ago, to the many many young people I have worked with since, I have always been driven by the desire to listen and to affirm. As such, writing this book is certainly not the end point of my journey of learning: I learn with every young person who shares part of their life with me. But in putting up my hand to write this book, I did so from a place of knowing. Not of knowing everything, but of knowing that some of the insights I have gained from the young people I work with, and how they challenge both public and clinical representations of transgender people, are important to share.

Writing this book, then, was very much a labour of love. It was a true intertwining of my own journey within critical psychology, and the journey I have undertaken with the many young people I have worked with. As a field of psychology, critical psychology seeks to challenge social norms, to examine how power operates to both privilege and marginalise, and to be liberatory in the sense of opening up new vistas for thinking about subjectivity. As children, as people, and as active agents in the world around them, the young people I have worked with push the remit of critical psychology to new ends by asserting themselves in the face of cisgenderism, by speaking to power from a place of knowing, and in so doing creating new vistas within which they and others (including myself) can think about gender.

Just as this book was informed by a simple premise, my approach to writing this book was simple. I sought to bring together two forms of evidence: the fictionalized (though not fictional) narratives of some of the young people I work with, and the latest research about transgender young people and their families. In so doing my goal was to challenge much of the received 'wisdom' that circulates about transgender young people, not by engaging in unnecessary critiques of previous literature, or by giving space to the voices of those who oppose transgender young people and their families, but rather by using a critical psychological lens through which to situate clinical practice with transgender young people and their families. This meant that whilst I am fully aware of literature that seeks to challenge or question transgender people's gender, it did not have much of a place in this book.

By staying away for the most part from aspects of the literature and public narratives about transgender people that often leave us 'stuck' in cisgenderism, I was able to write a book that is both situated and optimistic. It is situated in the sense that it is situated in the context of transgender young people's lives, and particularly their need for affirming clinical care. And it is situated in a literature that seeks to understand the specificities of transgender young people's lives. Importantly, this does not mean that the book shies away from debate when necessary. The situatedness that I adopted within this book, however, means that the debates that I engage with are never about the veracity of transgender young people's lives. Instead, any debates that I take up within this book challenge the terms of the debates themselves (i.e., the idea that transgender young people should be a topic of debate).

Focusing primarily on the lives of transgender young people and their families, then, allowed me to focus on topics that are often left to one side when debates over transgender young people predominate. Primarily it allowed me to think through what a critical developmental approach to working with transgender young people might look like. Mindful of the critical psychological deconstruction of 'developmentalism' (i.e., the idea that there is one 'correct' developmental pathway for all children), I was able to reconstruct an account of transgender young people's gender development, an account that emphasises diversity, that is both non-linear and non-normative, and which is grounded in a critical account of the latest literature in the field. Placing this alongside fictionalized case studies enabled me to provide an overview of the broad contours of gender development for transgender young people, without being prescriptive.

To frame my thoughts about gender development I generated a mnemonic that, in both my own clinical practice and that of other clinicians who have undertaken training with me, enables transgender young people's diverse journeys to be heard and engaged with. Eschewing diagnosis, the mnemonic is situated within an extended family context, and is mindful of the negative impact of cisgenderism upon all people. This situatedness and mindfulness means, I believe, that the GENDER mnemonic I outline in this book offers a critical psychological account of how to go about the work of adopting an affirmative approach to working with transgender young people. It most certainly owes more than a debt of gratitude to all of the scholars and clinicians who have advocated for affirming approaches, and who have made it possible for me to write this particular book. But it also builds upon this work, offering new avenues for thinking about how clinicians can best work with transgender young people through a lens that is critical of received wisdom, instead centring the knowledges that transgender young people bring with them to the clinical encounter.

Importantly, and as I noted above, the GENDER mnemonic is not prescriptive. There is no requirement that aspects of the mnemonic be addressed in any particular order, nor that any one aspect *must* be of relevance to a particular young person and their family. In other words, the mnemonic is *not* intended as yet another form of gatekeeping, and thus should *not* be used to keep transgender young people in a holding pattern controlled by the clinician. Instead, its utility is its capacity to open up productive conversations, but whether or not these are productive or simply not relevant can only be determined by young people themselves. This will mean that at differing ages or in the context of differing life experiences certain aspects of the mnemonic will be more salient. Again, it is young people who 'activate' our focus as clinicians on certain aspects of the mnemonic, rather than clinicians dictating what aspects should be given concerted attention.

As I came to see, however, having written this book, nothing is ever quite as simple as the account above might suggest. I was very fortunate to receive critical feedback on this book from many people, including other clinicians, parents of transgender young people, and from transgender adults (acknowledging, of course, that these three categories overlap). Some of the changes that resulted from this feedback, and which I signal here, add necessary complexity to this book. Indeed, starting with the word 'complexity', I use it throughout this book to argue that clinicians working with transgender young people should not seek simplistic answers, and specifically to suggest that there is no one singular transgender narrative. This, however, is not to suggest that clinicians should situate 'complexity' *within* transgender young people. We are all complex people, whatever our gender may be. Rather, my aim as a clinician is always to listen to the diversity of narratives that any one person brings with them, instead of trying to produce one definitive account of their life. This is different, however, to demanding that transgender young people spend unnecessary amounts of time 'unpacking their gender'.

As I will clearly argue in this book, my starting place is always that young people know their gender. But like all of us, living as we do in a context of social norms that regulate what forms of gender expression are intelligible, in my experience it is helpful to encourage conversations about what gender means and looks like, for both young people and their parents. This is in *no way* about questioning anyone's gender, or suggesting that they should live their gender in a different way. Nor is it about suggesting in *any way* that parents are somehow 'responsible' for a child being transgender. Instead, by having complex and critical conversations about gender, my aim is always to help young people to understand that the way they express their gender is entirely a matter of their own determination, and that there are no set rules about being a particular gender. For parents, and particularly those who may be struggling to understand a child who is transgender, talking to them about their own gender is about helping them to understand that just as they experience their gender to be true, so do their children. As such, discussions about gender may or may not be salient, depending on the journey that young people and their parents are undertaking.

Another word that I use throughout this book (and indeed this preface) is 'critical'. As I have elaborated above, this draws from the field of critical psychology, and is critical in the sense of examining social norms, and offering a creative space in which to think differently about normative assumptions. As such, my use of the word 'critical' is in no way associated with so-called 'gender critical' approaches, which seek to reassert the normative assumption that assigned sex determines gender, and hence that transgender people do not exist. Indeed, a critical psychological account of gender would be highly suspicious of 'gender critical' approaches, and would seek to deconstruct the types of claims made in the name of such approaches. I do just such deconstructive work within this book, as I carefully unpack how gender development has been historically understood, and how it may more productively be understood from a critical developmental starting place that seeks to be affirming of transgender young people.

Also important to note is that this book is not a 'how to' guide. There are many such books already on the market, some of which I summarise in Chap. 1. I intentionally did not write a 'how to' guide, partly because there are already so many on the market, partly because they are often region-specific, and partly because they can date quite quickly as our critical understanding about the needs and lives of transgender young people grows. Instead, this book is a clinical book in that it takes a critical stance on existing empirical literature so as to clear the way to an inclusive and affirming account of gender development that can be used by clinicians across the world, and it does so by linking the account that I develop closely with fictionalized clinical case material. My hope is that such a linking will bring into being new ways of thinking about clinical work with transgender young people, ways that challenge gatekeeping, and which are instead founded upon the knowledges that transgender young people bring to the clinical space.

Finally, and this is a vital point, clinicians must know when we should step out. Certainly, some transgender young people may need ongoing support, particularly in the context of mental health concerns arising from the effects of cisgenderism. Other families may need ongoing support as parents work through their own struggles. And at certain key points in their lives transgender young people may need to re-engage with clinicians for support. But there will also be many transgender young people who simply need access to clinical services to achieve a particular aim, whether that be puberty suppression or hormone therapies. Such services should be available with minimum wait times, and without gatekeeping that serves to prolong the wait to achieve a particular aim. Clinicians thus need to know when to step out, always leaving the door open should new needs arise.

In conclusion, I hope that readers of this book will see the complexity in the simple way that I have approached writing this book. That my focus on an affirming approach that is critical of received wisdom is understood as one that can only be determined by young people and their families: only they can determine what counts as affirming, and what might be experienced as gatekeeping. As such, despite the complexity and criticality that I introduce throughout this book, my premise remains simple: clinicians must be guided by young people in terms of how they understand their gender, and the goal should always be to listen and affirm, never to question unnecessarily for our own edification.

Adelaide, SA, Australia   Damien W. Riggs

Acknowledgements

I begin by acknowledging the sovereignty of the Kaurna people, the First Nations people upon whose land I live and work.

This book has been a long time coming, and has benefited from input from many people with whom I have had in depth conversations about the topics contained within it. Thanks must go to Ruth Pearce for insightful suggestions when I was reviewing the literature on gender development and adolescence. Thanks to Shoshana Rosenberg and Georgie Swift for lengthy conversations about clinical work. Thanks to Gavi Ansara for his leadership in the field of cisgenderism studies, and his generous insights about how to translate research into practice. Thanks to Nik Taylor and Heather Fraser for encouraging me to think about the intersections of human and animal lives, which led to some of the material addressed in Chap. 5. Thanks to Jo Hirst for many early conversations that helped me to decide what to include in this book, and to FierceMum for later conversations that helped me to clarify how my work might be misread. A special thanks to Clare Bartholomaeus for our many collaborations that informed this book, and for her generous proof reading and indexing. Many thanks are also due to Joanna O'Neill and Grace Jackson, commissioning editors at Palgrave, for providing such generous support throughout the writing of this book, to Christina Richards for believing in this book from the onset, and to Lilith Saintclaire for providing the wonderful cover image.

I was fortunate to be able to present my thoughts about the GENDER mnemonic to several audiences in 2018: as part of a webinar series for the Australian Psychological Society, in a workshop with Heidi Jansen at the Australian Psychological Society Clinical College conference, in a workshop for the Australian Association of Family Therapy, and in a workshop for the Australian Psychological Society Educational and Developmental Psychologists College. Thanks to all attendees for such insightful and constructive feedback, and to Judith Gullifer, Helen Linder, Nina Levin, and Helen Broomhall for their kind invitations to run these events.

As always, I must thank the family with whom I live: Leo, Gary, Jayden, Liam, Damian, Jeremiah, Herman, Patience, and Mandy, for supporting me in my work, and for always accommodating me when I need to focus on writing. Special thanks to my mother Sharon for helping me to continue to see clients when Jeremiah came into our family. Finally, my heartfelt thanks go to the many transgender young people and families with whom I have worked over the past decade. This book would never have happened without your insights.

Contents

1 Introduction 1

2 Children and Gender Development 31

3 Challenges and Joys in Adolescence 57

4 Parent Journeys Through Cisgenderism 83

5 Siblings, Grandparents, and Animal Companions 105

6 Conclusion 123

Author Index 145

Subject Index 147

1

Introduction

For most of my career I have thought of myself as a scientist-practitioner. To me, this is exemplified by the intersections of my clinical work as a psychotherapist who specialises in working with transgender children and their families, and my role as an academic whose research primarily focuses on the lives of transgender people. This image of myself as a scientist-practitioner was formed through my training in the discipline of psychology, where the scientist-practitioner model is very much a taken for granted norm, and in which the search for 'truth' central. Yet as part of my formation as a psychoanalyst, the topic of what counts as 'truth' very much came under question. Coming into a relationship with one's unconscious, and indeed coming to authorise oneself as a clinician – as is central to Lacanian psychoanalysis – led me to question what it means to 'know'. Furthermore, coming to grapple with my own complex gender histories as a nominally cisgender (i.e., not transgender) man led me to question what it means to 'know' one's gender, and how, as a clinician, I can understand the gender of another.

This book represents an attempt at coming to terms with what it means to 'know' gender in the context of working with transgender young people and their families. To know, I will argue, is always partial, and always situated. This includes what it means to know as a clinician, what it means to know as a young person, and what it means to know as a family member. Each of these different groups make unique claims to knowledge about gender, and each set of claims brings its own set of truths that are intersecting, yet distinct. They are intersecting, as I will explore in greater detail below, in the sense that they are all formed in a broader context of discrimination and social norms perpetuated in relation to transgender people. Yet they are distinct, in the sense that such discrimination and norms play out in very specific ways, according to one's social location, and the authority that one is differentially accorded.

Clinician readers may reasonably ask, what it means for me to begin this book by questioning what it is that we can know about gender. How, it may be asked, can a clinician work with transgender young people and their families if they cannot truly 'know'? The astute reader may also question the ontological quandary that such issues of epistemology raise. If there is no pre-given 'truth' of gender, how may this potentially undermine the truth claims made by young people about their gender? In this opening chapter I explore these types of questions via a careful unpacking of what it means to know as a scientist-practitioner who works with transgender young people and their families. At its simplest, my argument is that if our knowing is guided by an understanding of young people as experts on their gender, then it can be firmly grounded in a very specific set of ontological claims. At the same time, however, and as the subsequent chapters in this book elaborate, a critical developmental approach to working with transgender young people and their families affords us the necessary epistemological lens through which to understand gender. Such a lens, one that I believe to be novel to this book, enables clinician readers from all walks (i.e., psychologists, social workers, counsellors, and psychiatrists) to have the capacity to truly hear a diverse range of ontological claims about gender.

In the sections that follow, I first unpack in greater detail what it means to be a scientist-practitioner who adopts a critical approach to both 'science' and 'gender'. Through a consideration of the histories of the term 'scientist-practitioner' I propose a framing of this role for clinicians as one that adopts a critical account of gender, one informed by a particular understanding of the individual and institutional discrimination directed towards transgender people. Having outlined this account, I then turn to consider how others have outlined the role of clinicians who work with transgender young people and their families, highlighting how my own approach intersects with yet also diverges from the accounts of others, specifically in terms of its developmental focus. With these divergences considered, I then introduce my own conceptual framework for clinical work, one that keeps 'gender' at the forefront, whilst being focused on unpacking its constitutive parts. The chapter then finishes by summarising the contents of this book, locating each within a relationship to the epistemological claims outlined in this introductory chapter.

Problematising the Scientist-Practitioner Model

Much has been written about the scientist-practitioner model in psychology, but in this section I draw primarily on the work of John, an Australian critical psychologist whose writing did much to unpack the problems inherent to the model as it has traditionally been understood. As John argues (1994), from its inception the scientist-practitioner model accepted as its basis the assumption that there are universal laws that govern individual behaviour. The role of the scientist-practitioner is thus to identify such laws and apply them in the treatment of individuals. As John argues, however, the idea of universal laws only makes sense if individual behaviours are seen as a 'natural' reflection of innate truths about individuals. Moreover, the naturalisation of universal laws positions the scientist-practitioner as an objective bystander, capable of observing laws *in situ*, and doing so free of personal bias or beliefs.

The problem faced by the scientist-practitioner when it comes to clinical work is the fact that any so-called universal laws identified on the basis of experimental research abstracted from the lives of actual people all too often fails to be effective. Whilst psychology has long positioned itself as an evidence-based discipline (and certainly psychology is not alone in this claim, with the mental health professions in general making similar claims), the problem for the clinician, then, is that too often the evidence-base is ill suited to clinical work. This is not to say that certain modalities, developed from research, are entirely inefficacious. Rather, it is to suggest that using research findings to inform practice also requires some sort of translation, so as to meet the need of individuals. And it is this translation – which always involves the clinician's own views, beliefs, and biases – that draws attention to the shortcomings of the scientist-practitioner model as it is traditionally understood. In other words, if clinicians engage in practices of translation that are always shaped by their own views, beliefs, and biases, then it is almost certainly the case that the evidence base upon which the practice is based is, to a certain degree, lost in translation.

Part of what is lost in translation, I would argue, is keeping open the space for a critical view of science. When the clinician draws upon 'evidence-based principles' derived from a normative understanding of science, they do so by reifying a particular view of science. This view of science, as John (1994) argued, is one based upon the assumption that researchers are objective interpreters of the 'natural' world. Science as it is produced by scientists is thus seen as free from bias. We know, of course, that this is never the case. Not only do scientists bring their own biases to bear upon the types of research questions they investigate, and the methods by which they investigate them, but the ways in which scientific research is understood by others always occurs in a cultural context, rather than a cultural vacuum. Having a critical view of science, as I will outline in the following sections, is vital to any understanding of the scientist-practitioner model.

Gender and the Scientist-Practitioner Model

In terms of the reification of scientific knowledge, 'gender' as a concept is a useful example. Historically, within psychological research gender was framed as 'sex differences', thus emphasising differences between people based on presumed-to-be physiological differences 'between the sexes' (Stewart and McDermott 2004). 'Females' as compared to 'males' were seen as having unique strengths and weaknesses that were a product of what was read as uniquely sexed physiologies, and these were then seen to translate into specific psychological differences that were presumed to be consistent and generalisable. In reality, this focus on difference served only to produce the very differences it was purported to be based on (Hare-Mustin and Marecek 1990). For example, based on the assumption that women were inherently weak, best suited to motherhood, and given to emotionality, research that sought to demonstrate the 'truth' of these assumptions did just that. Women for whom these assumptions were incorrect, or women for whom these assumptions were true only at one specific moment in time, disappeared as 'noise' via a focus on distinct categories of 'sex differences'.

Similarly lost in translation as a result of research on 'sex differences' was any attention to the lived experience of a person's gendered self, and the expectations placed upon individuals as a result of their assigned sex. The latter, in other words, was seen to trump the former. As a corrective to this, feminist psychologists sought to shift the focus from sex to gender, with the latter being understood as a set of normative understandings of how individuals should experience their assigned sex, understandings located within power dynamics where men's views and experiences are valued over those of women. This focus on gender as lived experience was an important corrective to research on 'sex differences', in that it eschewed the idea that one (of two) genders was inherently better than the other. Unfortunately, however, early feminist research to a certain degree remained mired in the assumption that gender reflected some sort of essential truth about individuals, hard-wired in many of the same ways as what were seen as physiological differences (Weisstein 1993). Whilst the incorporation of an analysis of power was a vital contribution of early feminist work, it nonetheless failed to move beyond an essentialist account of gender.

From the 1990s onwards, critical scholars have examined how gender as a construct is made sense of, indeed how it is produced, within specific cultural contexts. Such accounts, whilst acknowledging that in many such contexts gender is treated as a salient category, and one imbued with considerable regulatory power, that it is not an ahistorical entity that has always existed. This type of account moves us beyond simply challenging gender hierarchies, to instead question how gender itself is naturalised, and how 'sex differences' are made to matter on very specific terms.

Indeed, from a critical perspective it has been argued that rather than seeing particular types of bodies as producing gender categories, instead it is more accurate to see particular forms of categorisation as producing bodies that are seen as naturally attached to certain genders. This is not to deny that as individuals we typically have a very real and embodied sense of our gender. Rather, it is to suggest that this embodied sense of gender is produced within cultural contexts where 'having a gender' offers us access to particular, normative, realms of intelligibility.

To return to the scientist-practitioner model, then, first sex, and then gender, have been seen as 'variables' through which certain phenomena, treated as 'natural', are made sense of. Women are expected to respond better to certain clinical techniques, men to others. More broadly, as an inherently masculinist enterprise, science itself as it is normatively understood privileges values typically associated with men (i.e., abstraction, rationalism, objectivity). Science, then, as it forms the basis for the scientist-practitioner model, is steeped in normative understandings of gender. Certainly, other approaches to science, as I will elaborate below, are possible. Feminist philosophers have long unpacked the masculinism of science and advocated for other accounts of science that question its very foundations (Harding 1987). My concern, however, is with the degree to which such alternate accounts have filtered through to the scientist-practitioner model, or whether the scientist-practitioner model remains mired in a normative understanding of both science and gender.

Cisgenderism and the Scientist-Practitioner Model

The account I provided above of the normative understandings of science and gender that would seem inherent to the scientist-practitioner model are especially vexed in the context of clinical work with transgender young people and their families. To understand why this is so, we can usefully engage with the work of Ansara and colleagues (Ansara 2010, 2015; Ansara and Hegarty 2014; Blumer et al. 2013; Riggs et al. 2015), who have explored in detail the concept of 'cisgenderism', understood as the ideology that delegitimises people's own understandings of their genders and bodies. In the context of the scientist-practitioner model, cisgenderism takes many forms. It can involve research that questions transgender people's genders, and/or treats them as pathological. It can involve clinical assessment tools that position mental health professionals as able to 'diagnose' transgender people's gender, thus serving to maintain the role of mental health professionals as gatekeepers to services. Cisgenderism can also include the assumption by clinicians that there are only two genders. This can mean that whilst a clinician may be supportive of a person who is transgender, they may be less than supportive if the person's gender does not conform to one of two binary categories. Finally, cisgenderism shapes how clinicians understand or describe the lives of transgender people. This can include where clinicians misgender people (i.e., use pronouns associated with a person's assigned sex, rather than their gender), utilise language that reinforces the idea that one's gender should somehow 'match' or 'align' with one's assigned sex in a normative sense, or continue to use terminology that is outdated (i.e., 'transsexualism', 'transgenderism', or using transgender as a verb – 'transgendered' – rather than as an adjective).

In this book I propose that central to a critical account of both gender and the scientist-practitioner model must be an understanding of cisgenderism. Cisgenderism constitutes the discriminatory contexts that I referred to in the introduction to this chapter, contexts that shape which voices will be accorded authority, and which voices will be relegated to the margins. For example, whilst there is now a growing body of affirming evidence-based approaches to clinical work with transgender young people and their families, these approaches arguably constitute a very recent (though far from complete) paradigm shift. Returning to the work of John (1994), this would suggest that the field of clinical work as it pertains to transgender young people and their families can best be understood as paradigmatic, whereby for a considerable period of time one particular clinical approach dominated (i.e., one that was alternatingly 'curative' or 'cautious' – see below), but where current research demonstrates that such approaches failed the 'do no harm' mandate. As a result, a new affirming paradigm is on the rise, though has most certainly been met with considerable resistance.

Claims to 'science' producing an 'evidence-base' about gender thus require considerable caution. Such a statement, of course, can as easily be applied to current affirming approaches as it can be applied to past approaches that were either 'curative' (i.e., attempting to enforce the assumption that a child's assigned sex should normatively determine their gender) or 'cautious' (i.e., adopting a 'wait and see' approach, rather than affirming young children in their gender). The difference that I will be arguing throughout this book is that the evidence base for the latter approaches were premised upon an uncritical view of science as reporting 'natural phenomena' (where gender binaries and gender as normatively determined by assigned sex were treated as 'natural'), in addition to the fact that they were rarely premised on the diverse views of young people with regard to gender. The more recent affirming approaches, though not necessarily any more critical of science as an enterprise more broadly, are most certainly critical of received knowledge about gender, and most certainly emphasise the importance of listening to young people's voices.

Being a Critical Scientist-Practitioner of Gender

To be a critical scientist-practitioner when working with transgender young people and their families, then, is greatly benefited by the four aspects of clinical practice outlined by John (1994), each of which can assist us in being mindful and critical of cisgenderism. The first involves 'knowing in action'. This pertains to clinicians having a clear understanding of cisgenderism and its impact upon transgender young people and their families. The second involves 'reflection in action'. This involves reflecting as one takes action, to ensure that one's understanding in the moment is in line with the client's understanding (so, for example, ensuring that one's own understanding of gender accords with that of one's client). The third involves 'reflecting on reflection in action'. By this, John refers to the need to go beyond moment-by-moment reflection that is always reactive, to develop from one's reflections an explicit account that can be applied in the future. Finally, John suggests the need for ongoing reflection on the explicit accounts that we derive from our reflection in action. Here John refers to the need for clinicians to constantly hone their knowledge, taking into account conflicting or new information, rather than attempting to arrive at a final and fixed account.

This book in many ways is an application of the third and fourth points made by John (1994). My clinical work as a scientist-practitioner has come from a form of knowing in action, one that continues to grow via my own critical reflection and learning. In reflecting upon my own reflection in action, I have been able to see common themes that repeat across clients, and which suggest a number of key strategies that I believe are central to an affirming approach to working with transgender young people and their families, and specifically one that aims to offer a critical approach to understanding gender development. This reflection has enabled me to develop an explicit account of my clinical work that is outlined later in this chapter and further in Chap. 2, however this account is open to ongoing reflection and revision. As such, the account that I provide below should not be taken as a definitive account of affirming practice. Rather, it should be a springboard for further developments, particularly those that arise from the voices of young people.

A critical affirming approach encompassing of gender development as employed by the scientist-practitioner is thus one that takes responsibility for ongoing cisgenderism within the mental health professions. It is one that views young people as experts on their gender, though this does not mean that clinicians should eschew developing their own knowledge: young people are not here to educate us, even if, when it comes to their gender, they are the experts. A critical affirming approach is also one that actively challenges social norms, rather than accepting them or taking them for granted. As Edwards-Leeper (2017) notes: "affirmative care values one's long-term psychological health and quality of life over maintaining the status quo as it relates to gender" (p. 123). For the scientist-practitioner, this means being willing to challenge received scientific knowledge, and indeed challenging the scientific endeavour itself as a meaning-making enterprise. The same is true with regard to gender. Whilst a critical affirming approach views young people as experts on their gender, this does not mean that clinicians cannot be critical of 'gender' as a category, and particularly with regard to its regulatory functions.

Further, it does not mean that clinicians cannot have a critical developmental account of gender that guides their practice, as will be outlined further in this chapter and in the chapters to come.

With regard to both 'science' and 'gender', then, a critical approach draws upon understandings of both that affirm an existing worldview (i.e., that advocating for the affirmation of transgender young people is vital), rather than necessarily deriving the worldview from normative accounts of science or gender. Such an approach is necessary given that, whilst as I suggested above drawing on the work of John (1994), we are witnessing a paradigmatic shift in clinical approaches to working with transgender young people and their families, such a shift is arguably driven less by science, and more by an ethics of care that recognises the damage done by past approaches. Certainly, science has a role to play in evidencing such damage, but we do not need scientific evidence to know that damage occurs. Rather, we listen to the voices of young people who inform us about our 'missteps', which Mizock and Lundquist (2016) suggest involve (1) expecting that transgender people educate clinicians, (2) making everything about gender, (3) having a narrow – potentially binary – understanding of gender, (4) avoiding talking about gender, (5) making generalisations about 'all transgender people', (6) seeing gender as something to be 'repaired', (7) pathologising transgender people's gender, and (8) gatekeeping access to services. Without suggesting that affirming clinicians never fall foul of these types of missteps, it is reasonable to suggest that they are most indicative of 'curative' or 'cautious' approaches that are still used by some clinicians, to the disbenefit of their clients.

Importantly, then, the approach I advocate for in this book is not an *ad hoc* approach comprised simply of practice wisdom developed on the fly. Rather, it is one driven by an overarching principle – that affirming approaches are both socially just and are enactments of a do no harm approach. Furthermore, it is an approach informed by a critical understanding of science and gender that values the intersections of academic research and theorising and clinical knowledge, whilst always appreciating that normative accounts of science, gender, and 'best practice' have at times been part of the problem.

Existing Approaches to Working with Transgender Young People and Their Families

In this section I provide a critical commentary on existing affirmative accounts of clinical work with transgender young people and their families. Importantly, all of the accounts that I cover are affirmative, and thus provide an important counter to previous approaches. Also important to recognise is that the accounts I examine run the gamut of peer reviewed academic research, popular books written for parents of transgender children (but which include a clinical focus), and instructional texts written for clinicians. These are thus a diverse collection of texts that are unified primarily by their adoption of an affirmative approach. In my reading of these texts, my focus is on how they account for science, whether or not their account of science includes a specific focus on cisgenderism, and how they account for gender development. My intention in undertaking this reading is not to discredit these texts so that I can posit my own account as inherently better. To do so would be to re-enact the traditional, masculinist, scientist-practitioner role, where science is always an 'up the hill' endeavour, built upon the bones of vanquished foes. Rather, my intention is to acknowledge where my approach aligns with existing affirming approaches, and where it offers something different.

A key early affirming text was *Transgender emergence* by Lev (2004). Lev's work has been at the forefront of advocating for an affirmative approach to working with transgender people and their families, though in this specific text Lev does not focus solely on children. In the text Lev does engage with what were then standard forms of 'diagnosis' with regard to transgender people, though it is important to be mindful of the time at which Lev wrote her book, a time where affirming approaches were very much at the margins. That she framed some of her text through the lens of normatively accepted tenets for diagnosis is thus understandable. Further, and despite any emphasis on diagnosis, Lev provides a thorough deconstruction of discrimination directed towards transgender people, albeit not through the lens of cisgenderism. Finally, and the strength of the text, is the affirming approach that Lev advocates for. As a clinical social worker, Lev (2004) emphasised an 'advocacy-based treatment modality' (p. 185), one that prioritises transgender people's right to self-determination, right to make informed decisions, and right to services. Such a modality, Lev suggests, may be usefully understood through the metaphor of 'therapist as midwife' (p. 221): "It is an evocative process in which the therapist is the midwife, assisting in the birthing, offering encouragement and support but essentially witnessing the client's own birthing process" (p. 223). On the basis of undertaking such a role, Lev proposes a stage model of 'transgender emergence'. Such stage models have been widely critiqued on the basis of their developmentalism (an issue I will explore in more detail in Chap. 2). More broadly speaking, stage models as applied to transgender are not developmental in terms of focusing on gender, but rather are developmental in terms of what is framed as a 'transgender identity'. My approach in this book in terms of gender development is considerably different, in that it attempts to map out a critical approach to understanding gender development for transgender young people.

Similarly written from a social work perspective, Mallon's (2009) edited collection *Social work practice with transgender and gender variant youth* emphasises an ecological approach to working with transgender young people. Such an approach focuses on the interaction between the individual and their environment, though in this text cisgenderism as environment is not given specific attention. Science as a meaning-making enterprise is depicted more holistically than the standard masculinist enterprise, with Mallon suggesting that clinicians should draw knowledge from practice wisdom (so a version of John's 1994, 'reflection in action'), history and current events, professional literature, empirical research and theories, and information provided by the client themselves. In this text gender is not critically theorised, though there certainly is a sense in which the authors appear to appreciate that binary models of gender are insufficient. Finally, whilst the book examines transgender young people's lives across a series of developmental periods, gender development itself is not theorised.

Of the peer-reviewed texts included in this section, Menvielle and colleagues (Hill and Menvielle 2009; Hill et al. 2010; Menvielle 2012) are among some of the most well-known advocates of an affirming approach, first undertaken as part of the *Children's Gender and Sexual Advocacy and Education Program,* and more latterly as the *Gender Development Program.* Their approach includes a primary focus on parents, including psychoeducation of parents, and peer-led support groups. In terms of clinical outcomes, the young people who attend their programme report higher rates of wellbeing as compared to young people who attend other, arguably less affirming, programmes. This would appear to be a result of the fact that the program helps to foster an affirming family environment for transgender children. Within the published materials about the programme, little mention is made of a critique of broader discrimination (and specifically cisgenderism) beyond the family, a critical account of gender does not appear to be evident (and the account of gender provided is not developmental in focus), and to date published materials have emphasised parents', as opposed to children's, voices.

The 'multi-dimensional family approach' advocated for by Malpas (2011) similarly views parents as "pillars of this therapeutic model" (p. 457). Different to the published accounts of the programme run by Menvielle and colleagues, however, Malpas includes a focus on working with parents to unpack how they understand gender as a concept. Similar to Menvielle and colleagues, Malpas emphasises research evidence as central to the affirming clinical endeavour, leaving little space for a critical examination of the role of 'evidence' in the perpetuation of cisgenderism. Gender as a category is largely taken for granted in the approach outlined by Malpas, with little critical attention to gender development amongst transgender young people.

Written specifically for parents (though with a sub-focus on clinicians), it is understandable that the 'conscious parenting' approach advocated for by Tando (2016) also focuses primarily on the role of parents. Importantly, however, Tando clearly emphasises the importance of viewing children as experts on their own gender, and does so through highlighting the difference between behaviour and being. Whilst not framed as a critical account of gender, in practice this focus on gender as 'being' rather than behaviour is an important corrective to approaches that would view transgender children as 'going through a phase'. Treating gender as 'being', of course, brings with it specific ontological issues, primarily that gender development amongst transgender children is not theorised (so there is a sense in the text that transgender children – or indeed all children – simply are a given gender, with no unpacking of how they come to understand their gender). Nonetheless, Tando does emphasise an affirming approach to a diversity of genders, rather than treating gender as a binary category. Building on this, Tando encourages parents to reflect on their own biases and understandings of gender, and in so doing directs readers to question received knowledge about gender. Whilst not framed through an understanding of cisgenderism, the text nonetheless encourages a critical stance towards gender norms, and assumptions about any presumed relationship between assigned sex and gender.

Of all of the texts, Tilsen's (2013) *Therapeutic conversations with queer youth: Transcending homonormativity and constructing preferred identities* provides the most thorough-going theoretical account of gender and social norms. Whilst not framed through the lens of cisgenderism, it nonetheless questions 'transnormativity', arguing that affirming approaches that only emphasise binary genders will always fail to meet the needs of all young people. Tilsen also critiques received understandings of science through an application of queer theory. Tilsen suggests that decentring professional knowledge is vital in order to create a space where young people can be heard on their own terms. As I will explore more in Chap. 2, this includes a critique of developmentalism, and its role in depicting young people as not mature enough to be experts on their own gender. Whilst a queer theory approach may not always be best suited for specific application to transgender young people (given that Ansara and Hegarty 2014, point to 'coercive queering' as a form of cisgenderism, i.e. that it should not be presumed transgender people are queer), it nonetheless provides a critical framework through which to theorise gender. Yet, given Tilsen's critique of developmentalism, gender development for transgender young people is not attended to within the text.

Within both parent and professional communities, two of the most well-known texts are written by Ehrensaft (2011a, 2016). A developmental and clinical psychologist, Ehrensaft has a long history of working with transgender young people, and has been a very strong advocate for affirming approaches. In her first text *Gender born, gender made* (2011a), Ehrensaft placed greater emphasis on working 'behind the scenes' with parents so as to equip them with skills and knowledge to affirm their child. In her second text *The gender creative child* (2016), however, Ehrensaft places much greater emphasis on children as experts on their own genders. Similarly, whilst in the first text Ehrensaft emphasis the utility of working cautiously (though nonetheless affirmingly) with young transgender people, in the second text Ehrensaft emphasises a more proactive approach, where the clinician as 'translator' "tak[es] in information from the child and family to reflect back what we see as the child's gender web" (p. 163). In both texts Ehrensaft is highly critical of received scientific knowledge about gender, and in the second text clearly locates high rates of poor mental health amongst transgender young people as a product of discrimination. Whilst such discrimination is not theorised as cisgenderism, Ehrensaft's 'gender creative' approach very much sees gender as diverse, rather than binary. At the same time, however, Ehrensaft's focus on the 'true gender self' with regard to transgender young people means that little space is given to unpacking gender development in the context of transgender young people's lives (i.e., when gender itself is taken as an ontological 'truth', this can tend to mitigate attention to gender as an epistemological category, particularly in terms of development). In other writings Ehrensaft (e.g., 2011b, 2012) has engaged to a certain degree with gender development for transgender young people, however in this work she primarily emphasises a kernel of 'truth' about gender evident at birth that is shaped both by internal physiological characteristics (such as in utero hormones) and by the world around. As such, even when acknowledging 'external forces', Ehrensaft emphasises a 'truth' about gender that pre-exists language (an issue I explore in more detail in Chap. 2).

Of the texts examined here, the one that is least critical of both gender and science is *Counseling transgender and non-binary youth: An essential guide* by Krieger (2017). Written for clinicians, there is a sense in which the text understands gender as something of a problem for transgender young people, as indicated by the focus on clinical evaluation as including sense of self, group affiliation, body discomfort, and regard by others. These areas of focus are not located within a broader context of cisgenderism, through which I would argue all four are produced. Nor are they viewed through a developmental lens in terms of gender (but instead, in a sense, are seen as problems of gender specific to transgender young people). Additionally, the text suggests that clinicians should "aim to be on everyone's side" (p. 149), so that parents do not perceive clinicians as biased towards children. As we shall see below, and as is indicated in many of the texts included in this section, whilst encouraging parents to be affirming can require delicate negotiations on the part of the clinician, this need not mean that clinicians should align themselves with parents and children equally.

Finally, *Transgender children and youth: Cultivating pride and joy with families in transition* by Nealy (2017) provides an important corrective to an affirming canon writing primarily by cisgender people (the present book included). As a clinical social worker and transgender man, Nealy writes from both standpoints in order to clearly outline an affirming approach to working with transgender young people. Nealy advocates for an expansive account of gender, and emphasises the importance of hearing the meaning that young people attribute to their genders, rather than focusing on 'why' or 'how' they are transgender. Whilst the text does not incorporate the cisgenderism framework, a critical account of the scientific enterprise, nor a developmental account of gender (though it certainly looks at gender across the lifespan), it most certainly situates clinicians within broader discriminatory contexts, and cautions clinicians to be aware of our own biases.

In sum, and bearing in mind the arguments I have made previously in this chapter, few of the texts summarised above include a thorough going critical analysis of gender or science, though most are cognisant of the role of science in producing normative understandings of gender, and most centre an understanding of gender that does not over-emphasise binary categories. In terms of cisgenderism as a framework, none of the books utilise this approach, however most are cognisant of the effects of discrimination, and its role in shaping the experiences of young people, their families, and clinicians. Finally, whilst some of the books touch on developmental issues, or include a lifespan focus, they do not offer a critical conceptualisation of gender development for transgender young people. Again, it is important to reiterate that these are a diverse collection of books written for diverse audiences. As such, the overview above is simply that: it situates the present book within a broad and diverse field, rather than seeking to highlight limitations in order to justify the present book. If anything, as we shall see below, there are some common themes in these other texts that are included in the present text, even if framed in different ways. And this is as it should be: an affirming approach that treats children as experts on their genders will always be unified by this view, even if each specific iteration will enact this in differing ways.

The GENDER Mnemonic

As I noted above, the approach that I take to affirming clinical work with transgender young people and their families bears many similarities to the work summarised above. It views children as experts on their gender. It views gender as more than two binary categories. It eschews diagnosis in favour of meaningful dialogue with young people and their families. It does not see therapy as an essential requirement for all transgender young people, though it acknowledges that many young people benefit from talking about their gender and how it is understood by the world around them. It is highly critical of developmentalism. Relatedly, it most certainly views parents as allies in the affirming process, though does not treat parents' views as the most important. These are widely accepted tenets of affirming approaches, and form the basis for the approach that I adopt in my own clinical work.

Where my approach adds additional dimensions is twofold. The first is through a focus on cisgenderism as playing a causative role in terms of the challenges faced by many transgender young people and their families. This can include where parents narrate their child's journey as a 'loss', a topic that I will explore in more detail in Chap. 4. Cisgenderism can also play a role in young people's experiences of dysphoria, a point that colleagues and I have made more broadly in terms of understanding factors associated with poor mental health amongst transgender people (Riggs et al. 2015). Cisgenderism shapes institutional responses to transgender young people and their families, particularly in schools, as Clare Bartholomaeus and I have elsewhere examined (Bartholomaeus and Riggs 2017). And as I will explore in Chap. 5, cisgenderism can be a tool that siblings and other family members use to control transgender young people. Speaking about cisgenderism with young people and their families thus offers a useful lens through which to understand discrimination directed towards transgender people, and to proactively identify moments where it is likely to occur.

My approach, as outlined already in this chapter, also includes a critical focus on both science and gender development. As we shall see in the chapters to come, there are certainly instances where I refer to the empirical literature when working with young people and their families. But in my clinical work I also provide young people and their families with critical interpretations of the literature. Both young people and parents are often well aware of published literature, having undertaken Internet searches before coming to see me. Providing critical insights about the limitations of existing research, its biases, and its at times unfounded claims often helps young people and their parents to adopt a more critical stance towards science, and can help engender a shift towards parents seeing their children as experts on their gender. In terms of gender, I strongly believe that an affirming approach should not eschew a focus on gender. It is all too easy to posit that viewing children as experts on their gender means that we cannot talk to children about their gender. Given that normative stereotypes about gender circulate, it is unsurprising that many transgender young people wholeheartedly adopt available gender norms, as is true for most people. My role as I see it is not to critique their gender presentation, but rather to bring awareness to the diverse ways that people live their gender, so that young people have a critical lens through which to view gender. This is something that I believe *all* people can benefit from, not simply transgender young people.

The twofold additional dimensions that this book brings to the existing affirmative literature can be usefully framed through a mnemonic that uses 'GENDER' as its acronym. For those working in the field and who adopt an affirming approach, this mnemonic is intended as a tool for case formulation, not a tool for 'diagnosis'. Its role is to help clinicians in working through some of the key issues that transgender young people and their families may often experience, and to ensure that families are adequately supported. It is not prescriptive, and as I noted above, is not intended to be closed off from revision. Rather, like Lev's (2004) account of 'transgender emergence', or Ehrensaft's (2011a, b, 2016) account of 'gender creative' children, it open to change, to extension, and to development. With these points in mind, I know outline the mnemonic, which is constituted by:

- **G**ender journey and understanding
- **E**xpressed concerns
- **N**ecessary actions
- **D**istress management
- **E**cologies of support
- **R**einforcement and resistance

Gender Journey and Understanding

It is important to reiterate from the onset with regard to this first part of the mnemonic, that our goal as clinicians is never to ask young people how they know that they are transgender, or why they are transgender, or how they know the truth of their gender. Parents will often offer anecdotes that function to answer these types of questions, but it is important to always emphasise that children's accounts of their gender are our starting and ending place, even if at times it will be useful to locate their gender within a critical developmental framework *that is inclusive of transgender young people*. As such, speaking with a young person about their gender journey is about learning what their gender *means* to them. Certainly, some of the information provided will usefully inform a psychosocial history, but more broadly it is an opportunity for young people to speak about what gender means to them as a category, how they live their gender, what they see for themselves from the future in terms of their gender, and how they situate themselves in terms of the category 'transgender'. These conversations should always be undertaken in ways appropriate to the child, their life experiences, their current needs, and their capacity to think through gender as a category.

For (primarily cisgender) parents, focusing on their own gender journeys and understandings can be a useful way of identifying barriers to parents affirming their children, including their own biases, fears, and worries about impression management when it comes to other people. Asking parents to reflect on how they understand their own gender, as well as gender as a category (i.e., do they see it as an immutable part of nature or as a cultural construct), can often help parents to understand that their child's gender is 'real': that it reflects their own lived truth. Reflecting on their own childhood can help parents to identify the impact of gender norms, and to have understanding for their child's experiences. As parents share their own views, this also offers opportunities to challenge gender stereotypes, and to reflect back to both parents and young people other ways of understanding gender. Framing their own accounts of their gender through a developmental lens also helps to draw out similarities between their own gender development and that of their children. Importantly, however, focusing on how parents experience their own gender should never be about implying that parents 'make' their child transgender. Rather, it is about identifying potential barriers that some parents may experience to being affirming, and to finding pathways out of any barriers.

Expressed Concerns

As we know from the literature, many young transgender people come to see clinicians with concerns, particularly about the future. These may involve fears about bullying or discrimination, worries about puberty, a strong desire to commence hormone therapy, generalised anxiety that is often a product of broader cisgenderist social contexts, and worries about fitting in and acceptance at school. Many young people also speak about experiences of dysphoria, and some also speak about the feeling that their parents don't truly accept their gender. Certainly it is the case that not all young people have these (or other) concerns, and certainly as I noted above, therapy is not mandatory. But for many young people, identifying key 'sticking points' can help lead to strategies for responding to or managing concerns or distress. Importantly, expressed concerns may be unique to being transgender, or they may be part of a broader narrative of gender development experienced by most children. Sometimes the role of the clinician is to unpack the concerns to see what might be specific to being transgender, and what might be more broadly about their gender (and thus similar to other children of the same gender, even with unique inflections arising from how transgender people are viewed and treated).

A critical developmental approach, as I outline in more detail in Chap. 2, can thus be important for helping to unpack expressed concerns.

For parents, expressed concerns can overlap with those of young people, but they can also be markedly different. Parents may worry about whether they can 'truly know' what their child's gender is, and may seek a diagnosis as a means to reassurance. Parents may worry about what kind of life their child will have, a life that may differ from their own dreams for their child. Parents may speak about 'loss' with regard to their child's gender, or fears about how other people will view them (i.e., as being too liberal as parents if they affirm their child). Fathers may often struggle the most with affirming their child, instead holding onto normative understandings of sex and gender, though certainly mothers often struggle too. Identifying the concerns that parents have offers the opportunity for psychoeducation with regard to gender, including offering a critical account of gender development. Such a critical account of development, as I noted above, can help parents to understand how each of us comes to understand ourselves as gendered beings, without resorting to a simplistic account of gender as a truth that exists prior to birth.

Necessary Actions

For some young people, the necessary actions are few. Their parents are supportive, the journey ahead is clear, and they are content to enjoy their lives, with very minimal interaction with a clinician. For other young people, however, and particularly for those whose parents may be struggling, a raft of actions may be necessary. This can include support in changing their name and gender legally, support in social transition, support in accessing other services (such as for fertility preservation and puberty blockers), and advocacy to schools and other institutions. Certainly, even for children of supportive parents, some of this advocacy work in terms of necessary actions may still be necessary. I often say to parents 'we don't know what we don't know': many parents may not have thought about, for example, fertility preservation, or may have limited understanding of pathways to care. This may have nothing to do with not being supportive, and everything to do with not knowing where to turn, or what information to trust.

Stemming from these necessary actions, it is important for parents to understand the difference between a need and a want. Parenting involves knowing when it is okay to say no to a 'want', but that a need is a different category entirely. Similar to Tandos' (2016) differentiation between a behaviour and being, a need for transgender young people, if fulfilled, can be the difference between happiness and depression. Working with parents, as I will explore in detail in Chap. 4, in order to move ahead to address necessary actions, is often a core component of clinical work with transgender young people and their families.

Distress Management

For many transgender young people, expressed concerns can be accompanied by a significant degree of distress. Dysphoria is often a key form of distress, but it is certainly not the only form that distress can take. Distress can be influenced by a future-orientation, in which young people are focused on their hoped for future (often including puberty blockers and then hormone therapy), at the expense of focusing on the now. As such, distress management focused on the now can involve attention to strategies that help ameliorate or reduce dysphoria, as we will explore in Chap. 3. In short, whilst it is rarely clinically useful to try and minimise how significant distress can be, and especially dysphoria, there is also a key role for clinicians to creatively negotiate ways to ensure that distress is not the only narrative available.

For parents, witnessing their child's distress can be very challenging. Working in collaboration with parents can often be vital to ensuring that any strategies aimed at addressing a young person's distress are put into action. As I will explore in detail in Chap. 4, parents can also experience distress of their own. This is often attached, as I suggested above, to their own dreams or hopes for their child, dreams or hopes that they may often feel disappear if their child is transgender. Working with parents to situate their dreams and hopes in a broader context of cisgenderism can be an important strategy to support them to re-narrate their expectations. If not, ongoing parental distress can be a barrier to their child being affirmed.

Ecologies of Support

I use the term 'ecologies of support' to recognise that support for transgender young people and their families can come from a diverse range of sources. Sometimes the most obvious forms of support are not available, or don't work for the young person. If this is the case, creative thinking is required to identify supports beyond those that may seem obvious. An ecological approach to support, then, means working with young people and their families, having identified expressed concerns and necessary actions, to recognise that many differing forms of support may be required, dependent on the need or distress. A peer support group, for example, may be beneficial for some young people. Yet if such a group is solely comprised of young people with a binary gender, will it be useful for a young person whose gender is non-binary? Again, focusing on ecologies of support means broadening our net so as to encompass the most diverse range of supports possible.

For parents, focusing on ecologies of support can include exploring sources that may at first appear supportive and affirming, but as time progresses may be less so. For example, extended family members who may initially appear supportive, but who over time continually misgender the young person. Parents too, then, need a diverse range of supports so that they are not overly reliant on one particular person or group or people who may be likely to bring with them their own biases.

Reinforcement and Resistance

Finally, as clinicians we have a clear role to play in using our epistemic authority to advocate for young people. This, at first glance, may seem to buy into the logic that adults know best, or that professionals know best. This is far from the case. Rather, the point about clinician reinforcement is that we can use received understandings of science to positive ends. We can make recourse to our clinical or academic knowledge to reinforce young people's views to their families. Whilst we will often do this alongside having a critical stance on science, this is not contradictory. Rather, it is about being accountable for the epistemic status we are accorded, which can comfortably sit alongside being critical of received knowledge that is not affirming. Modelling critical thinking to parents, for example, can encourage parents to be both affirming of their child, and critical of their own biases and those of others. In terms of resistance, this can involve acknowledging young people's agency, and the ways in which they resist normative framings of their lives. Acknowledging this and taking a lead from young people can constitute an important form of advocacy.

Reinforcement by the clinician also involves us taking a broader worldview on the lives of the young people we work with. Importantly, this is not a developmentalist claim. It is not to suggest that children cannot see their own lives in a holistic sense. Rather, it is to have the privilege of being able to take an outsider's vantage point, regardless of our own gender journeys. And it is this privileged perspective that can allow us to help young people and their families to situate their own journeys in a broader context. This can involve situating the challenges they face in a context of cisgenderism and to identify ways to challenge this. It can involve raising topics that the family may not have thought about (such as fertility preservation). In other words, alongside listening to children as experts on their gender, we should not eschew our own knowledges, and how they may be helpful. At the same time, and as I noted before, and as Ehrensaft (2011b) suggests, it is important that as clinicians we don't claim to know everything about gender. We must remain open to young people's agency, and to learn from the resistances that they raise to cisgenderism.

Chapter Overviews

As noted by the title of this book, my focus is on transgender young people. Specifically, my focus is on transgender young people who have a binary gender (i.e., male or female). In many ways this is problematic, given that central to an affirming approach, as outlined above, is recognition of a diversity of genders beyond binary categories. At the same time, however, I argue here that a critical developmental account of gender will look very different for young people with a binary gender as compared to young people with a non binary gender. Given the constraints of any book project, it seemed important to me not to do a disservice to any one group of young people by trying to be all inclusive. Rather, focusing solely on transgender young people with a binary gender has allowed me the necessary space to explore in depth their needs in a clinical context. Further, I am also aware from my clinical experience and from existing research that the experiences of young people who do not have a binary gender are often very different with regard to cisgenderism. In other words, cisgenderism does not uniformly affect everyone in the same way. It will impact upon non binary young people in very specific ways. I hope that in the near future a book will be published that focuses exclusively on non-binary young people (mirroring recent books that focus on non-binary adults: see Richards et al. 2017).

In terms of the contents of the chapters to follow, Chap. 2 focuses specifically on young children. It maps out a critical developmental account of gender, and in so doing challenges normative accounts that have been exclusionary or pathologising of transgender children. By examining the literature on early gender development I provide some epistemological leverage by (1) demonstrating how existing developmental accounts can actually be inclusive of transgender children, and (2) indicating where we need to go beyond existing accounts in order to be inclusive. This chapter is foundational in that it sets up a critical developmental account that follows through in subsequent chapters.

Chapter 3 then turns to consider transgender adolescents, and again considers the developmental literature for how it might already have the capacity to recognise and include transgender adolescents, but also key points where the developmental literature needs to shift its own boundaries and configurations in order to understand the specificities of puberty and adolescences for transgender young people. Considering topics such as fertility and intimacy, this chapter eschews the assumption often made that transgender adolescents must forgo loving relationships or plans for parenthood. Instead, this chapter advocates for what clinicians must attend to in order to ensure that transgender adolescents can experience all that is possible in their lives, and to do so safely and with support.

Chapter 4 attempts to grapple with what is often a difficult literature, namely the literature on parents of transgender children. This literature is difficult, I suggest, because so often it is weighed down in narratives of 'loss' that are presumed to shape the experiences of parents. By again utilising a developmental framework, I demonstrate how narratives of loss are produced by cisgenderism inherent both to developmental research, but also to normative assumptions about parenthood. Looking at how the two are intertwined allows me to consider how as clinicians we might move beyond narratives of loss to find ways to work with parents that celebrate their transgender children by taking a critical stance on assumptions about gender and parenting.

In offering a substantive focus on other family members (including grandparents, siblings, and animals), Chap. 5 broadens out the previous affirming literature on transgender young people to situate them in familial contexts broader than just parent-child relationships. In this chapter, and following the GENDER mnemonic focus on ecologies of support, I argue that a whole-of-family focus is vital if our aim as clinicians is to best support transgender young people. The focus on animals who live in the house is an especially important avenue of support that has rarely received attention in previous texts focused on transgender young people.

The final chapter of this book brings together the arguments made across the book with regard to gender, development, and what it means to be 'critical' as a scientist-practitioner. Specifically, it considers barriers to best practice including clinician attitudes and the contexts we practice in, how to work collaboratively with other clinicians to the benefit of transgender young people and their families, and the ways in which we can go about creating better worlds for the young people we work with. The chapter also returns to consider the GENDER mnemonic, demonstrating its efficacy in practice and avenues for its development in the future.

Concluding Thoughts

In this introductory chapter I have sought to develop a critical account of gender and science, one that views an understanding of cisgenderism as central to affirming clinical practice with transgender young people and their families. The account I have provided requires a constant weaving back and forth between an awareness of the epistemic authority accorded to clinicians as scientist-practitioners, and the need to be critical of received understandings of both science and gender. Similarly, it requires a constant weaving back and forth between a critique of developmentalism (as we shall explore in more detail in Chap. 2), and the utility of a critical developmental account of gender as it applies to transgender young people. Most certainly, this is at times a difficult tightrope to walk. To be affirming via reinforcement, for example, can all too easily slip into treating the scientist-practitioner as the 'expert'. Similarly, making recourse to developmental accounts can all too easily slip back into viewing such accounts as the sole 'truth' about gender. The task for the affirming clinician, then, is to continuously engage with John's (1994) injunction to act, reflect, and then to reflect some more.

In sum, the critical developmental approach that I advocate for in this book, as will be explored in greater detail in the chapters to come, is situated in a broader constellation of affirming approaches. The fictionalised clinical case materials that I present, and the focus on very specific constellations of journeys as elaborated through the GENDER mnemonic, will encourage readers to think more expansively about the work that they do, to focus on complexities rather than seeking simplistic solutions, and to know that the work we do is always situated in a broader social context that more often than not will *not* be affirming of our work. To be a critical clinician, then, is to take responsibility for the epistemic authority we are accorded, and to use this as a starting place from which to engage with transgender young people, their families, and the world around us.

References

Ansara, Y. G. (2010). Beyond cisgenderism: Counselling people with non-assigned gender identities. In L. Moon (Ed.), *Counselling ideologies: Queer challenges to heteronormativity* (pp. 167–200). Aldershot: Ashgate.

Ansara, Y. G. (2015). Challenging cisgenderism in the ageing and aged care sector: Meeting the needs of older people of trans and/or non-binary experience. *Australasian Journal on Ageing, 34*(S2), 14–18.

Ansara, Y. G., & Hegarty, P. (2014). Methodologies of misgendering: Recommendations for reducing cisgenderism in psychological research. *Feminism & Psychology, 24*(2), 259–270.

Bartholomaeus, C., & Riggs, D. W. (2017). *Transgender people and education.* New York: Palgrave Macmillan.

Blumer, M. L., Ansara, Y. G., & Watson, C. M. (2013). Cisgenderism in family therapy: How everyday clinical practices can delegitimize people's gender self-designations. *Journal of Family Psychotherapy, 24*(4), 267–285.

Edwards-Leeper, L. (2017). Affirmative care of TGNC children and adolescents. In A. A. Singh & l. m. dickey (Eds.), *Affirmative counseling and psychological practice with transgender and gender nonconforming clients* (pp. 119–142). Washington: American Psychological Association.

Ehrensaft, D. (2011a). *Gender born, gender made: Raising healthy gender-nonconforming children.* New York: The Experiment.

Ehrensaft, D. (2011b). Boys will be girls, girls will be boys: Children affect parents as parents affect children in gender nonconformity. *Psychoanalytic Psychology, 28*(4), 528.

Ehrensaft, D. (2012). From gender identity disorder to gender identity creativity: True gender self child therapy. *Journal of Homosexuality, 59*(3), 337–356.

Ehrensaft, D. (2016). *The gender creative child: Pathways for nurturing and supporting children who live outside gender boxes.* New York: The Experiment.

Harding, S. (1987). *The science question in feminism.* New York: Cornell University Press.

Hare-Mustin, R. T., & Marecek, J. (1990). *Making a difference: Psychology and the construction of gender.* Connecticut: Yale University Press.

Hill, D. B., & Menvielle, E. (2009). "You have to give them a place where they feel protected and safe and loved": The views of parents who have gender-variant children and adolescents. *Journal of LGBT Youth, 6*(2–3), 243–271.

Hill, D. B., Menvielle, E., Sica, K. M., & Johnson, A. (2010). An affirmative intervention for families with gender variant children: Parent ratings on child mental health and gender. *Journal of Sex & Marital Therapy, 36*(1), 1–18.

John, I. D. (1994). Constructing knowledge of psychological knowledge: Towards an epistemology for psychological practice. *Australian Psychologist, 29*(3), 158–163.

Krieger, I. (2017). *Counseling transgender and non-binary youth: An essential guide.* Philadelphia: Jessica Kingsley Publishers.

Lev, A. I. (2004). *Transgender emergence: Therapeutic guidelines for working with gender-variant people and their families.* New York: Haworth Press.

Mallon, G. P. (Ed.). (2009). *Social work practice with transgender and gender variant youth* (2nd ed.). New York: Routledge.

Malpas, J. (2011). Between pink and blue: A multi-dimensional family approach to gender nonconforming children and their families. *Family Process, 50*(4), 453–470.

Menvielle, E. (2012). A comprehensive program for children with gender variant behaviors and gender identity disorders. *Journal of Homosexuality, 59*(3), 357–368.
Mizock, L., & Lundquist, C. (2016). Missteps in psychotherapy with transgender clients: Promoting gender sensitivity in counseling and psychological practice. *Psychology of Sexual Orientation and Gender Diversity, 3*(2), 148–155.
Nealy, E. C. (2017). *Transgender children and youth: Cultivating pride and joy with families in transition.* New York: W. W. Norton and Company.
Richards, C., Bouman, W. P., & Barker, M. J. (Eds.). (2017). *Genderqueer and non-binary genders.* New York: Springer.
Riggs, D. W., Ansara, G. Y., & Treharne, G. J. (2015). An evidence-based model for understanding the mental health experiences of transgender Australians. *Australian Psychologist, 50*(1), 32–39.
Stewart, A. J., & McDermott, C. (2004). Gender in psychology. *Annual Review of Psychology, 55*, 519–544.
Tando, D. (2016). *The conscious parent's guide to gender identity.* Avon: Adams Media.
Tilsen, J. (2013). *Therapeutic conversations with queer youth: Transcending homonormativity and constructing preferred identities.* New York: Aronson.
Weisstein, N. (1993). Power, resistance and science: A call for a revitalized feminist psychology. *Feminism and Psychology, 3*(2), 239–245.

2

Children and Gender Development

Two questions are often at the forefront when I meet with parents of transgender children: How can *I* be sure about my child's gender, and how is my *child* sure about their gender. As I will explore in this chapter, the first question is one that can be construed as a question about aetiology. The second question is one that pertains to child development. As we shall see in this chapter, in many ways transgender children bring to light important questions about current understandings of gender development. Importantly, my suggestion here is not that transgender children should be a testing ground for gender theories. Rather, my point is that without even knowing it, existing theories of gender development already speak to the lives of transgender children, they just require some careful unpacking in order to be seen as applicable to the lives of transgender children.

At the same time, however, it would be too simple to just 'clarify' existing theories and the space they may provide for transgender children's understandings of their gender. Also needed is an examination of the normativity inherent in existing theories, as well as in existing clinical accounts of transgender children. This is in line with the specific affirming approach that I outlined in the first chapter of this book, which

© The Author(s) 2019
D. W. Riggs, *Working with Transgender Young People and their Families*, Critical and Applied Approaches in Sexuality, Gender and Identity,
https://doi.org/10.1007/978-3-030-14231-5_2

advocates for mental health professionals as scientist-practitioners taking a critical developmental approach to our understandings of gender. As such, in this chapter I first explore accounts of early acquisition of gender as a cognitive category, mapping how, far from being applicable only to cisgender children, such accounts are in fact a clear argument for the veracity of transgender children's understandings of their gender. Having provided this overview, I then turn to consider how, despite the space that already exists for including transgender children in developmental accounts of gender, cisgenderism functions to largely exclude transgender children from the realms of normative gender acquisition. With this critique in mind, I then consider how cisgenderism and developmentalism shape the diagnostic tools that are typically used by clinicians working with transgender children.

'Learning Gender', 'Knowing Self'

As I noted at the beginning of this chapter, parents often want to know how they can be sure about their child's gender, and to a certain degree this is a distinct question from how their child knows about their own gender. I suggest these are distinct questions because, faced with a child who has clearly asserted their gender, many parents can, to varying degrees, accept that this is how their child understands themselves. But given the cultural propensity to place under suspicion the beliefs and values that children hold, it is not automatic that a child's expression of their gender will be enough evidence for a parent to accept that their child knows of what they speak. As I outlined in Chap. 1, our starting place for an affirming approach to working with transgender children is that children are experts on their gender, but in many ways this runs counter to cultural scripts that view children as experts on very little, and certainly not something as important as their gender.

Given this chapter focuses on children, as distinct from Chap. 3 which focuses on adolescents, it is conceptually useful in this chapter to begin with very young children, as the youngest of children are often those most likely to be subjected to disbelief from their parents. Whilst in my own clinical experience the youngest child I have worked with was aged three (and her parents were very accepting and affirming), in many cases I often find out that the slightly older children I see (specifically a relatively large cohort of seven year olds) have been expressing their gender to their parents since they could speak, but their parents dismissed their expressions. One reason for this, as we shall explore in the following section, pertains to accepted wisdom about children's ability to understand gender, and the ages at which this occurs. Yet as I will now outline, research has increasingly suggested that children categorise people (including themselves) on the basis of what we as adults would understand as 'gender' from a much younger age than is widely understood.

Before considering what the research has to say on infants and gender, it is very important to first draw attention to what I see as a slippage in the literature. In their summary of cognitive theories of gender development, for example, Martin, Ruble and Szkrybalo (2002) refer to research demonstrating that "infants do hold gender categories in mind for at least some time, rather than forming them ad hoc" (p. 919). I would suggest caution is required with regard to this interpretation of the literature, particularly with regard to the term 'gender categories'. The literature on cognitive development is unilaterally clear that children from birth (and indeed perhaps *in utero*) can discern different categories of a given phenomenon. This might include different temperatures, different volumes of noise, different vocal tonalities, and different smells. Cognitively very young children are able to sort the differences they encounter into categories, though as Fausto-Sterling (2012) notes with regard to gender, these categories will likely be shades of grey, rather than black and white.

This point about shades of grey is central to how we apprehend early understandings of gender, as is the point above about categories. To render this another way: there is no doubt that from early infancy onwards, most children can sort people into groupings, though it is likely those groupings will be relatively flexible and open to new information should the boundaries of any grouping require resorting. Furthermore, the groupings that very young children make are done absent of access to verbal language. Given, then, that the cognitive structures that are involved in the grouping of people is not yet attached to language, to say that children understand 'gender categories' is to impute linguistic meaning to a system of categorisation not based on language. Can very young children potentially group all adults they encounter with relatively higher voices, for example, into one broad group, and all people with relatively lower voices into another broad group? Yes. But does that mean very young children then see those two groups as 'female' and 'male'? No.

The important question, then, is when does gender become a salient organising category that is labelled as such, rather than as a generic category comprised of groups not marked by gender as a construct? As I indicated above, and following Fausto-Sterling (2012), gender as an organising principle of categorisation likely comes into play with language. As children develop both receptive and expressive language, they are afforded means to linguistically organise the information they have been collecting about categories that we would understand as referencing gender. So, for example, if a child has developed a broad category that collects within it every adult they have interacted with who has a deeper voice, and as they enter into language they apprehend that every time one of these people are spoken about the pronoun 'he' is used, then that descriptor becomes attached to the category. This point about the linking of descriptors to categories is an important one. If infants have a range of categories that we would describe as referencing gender, but all they have available to them are two linguistic terms through which to sort the categories (i.e., she or he), then this drastically narrows the ways in which the categories are understood. What were likely grey categories that may (in reference to what adults would call 'gender') have been expansive and very likely greater in number than just two categories, become narrowed down through language. As the research summarised in the following section would seem to suggest, it is here that cisgenderism, at a very young age, comes to shape children's understandings of gender, limiting it to a binary system.

There is, however, another important limitation inherent to how children come to attach linguistic descriptors to cognitive categories. Specifically with regard to gender, most children do not include in their categorisation schema a visual inspection of genitalia – they are typically not privy to this information. Yet much of the literature on children and early understandings of gender draws a false equivalence between assigned sex and gender in terms of children's understandings. Here I want to suggest that we need to discard the assumption that what very young children know about gender directly references assigned sex, either their own or that of others. Rather, what children know about gender pertains to a system of categorisation developed pre-verbally that is then narrowed down through the acquisition of language, and only later becomes normatively attached to cisgenderist assumptions about genitalia and gender.

What does all of this mean for transgender children, and my promise in the introduction to this chapter that existing accounts of gender acquisition already speak to transgender children? In their summary of research on cognitive theories of gender development, Owen Blakemore, Berenbaum and Liben (2009) suggest that around the time that children begin to speak, they are also able to recognise themselves as distinct entities when looking in a mirror: distinct from other children and separate to their parent(s). This capacity to see oneself as an entity in one's own right means that the rules of categorisation that one has applied to other people then become applicable to oneself. In the box below the first aspect of the GENDER case formulation considers how one particular child speaks about her gender.

Case Study 1: Gender Journey and Understanding

Cara was eight when she first came to see me with her mother Amanda and her father Peter. Cara had two older siblings, Wendy and Chris. Cara was a very assertive and clearly spoken child who, despite her parents being somewhat hesitant in their support, had managed to negotiate to wear the clothes she wanted to wear (primarily by borrowing them from her sister), and was experiencing some success in getting her parents and siblings to call her Cara and use female pronouns.

At our first appointment Amanda and Peter were very keen that I undertake an assessment of Cara, so that they could be 'sure' that it would be the right thing to do to support Cara. My emphasis to the parents was that an assessment wouldn't be particularly useful given Cara's age, and that the best approach would be for us to just go with what Cara had to say. Taking that as her lead, Cara launched into a lengthy description of her gender, focusing on liking to have long hair, and enjoying playing with her sister's Barbie dolls. Amanda and Peter acknowledged that this was all very true, but countered that anyone could have long hair – indeed Amanda had short hair but was most certainly a woman – and that toys can be played with by anyone.

> I then asked Cara to speak more about what it means to be a girl. Cara then provided what turned out to be a very useful way of accounting for her gender. She said that 'being a girl feels natural, but being a boy would be random'. I asked Cara to unpack this last word, given that many children use the word 'random' to mean 'spontaneous' or 'unexpected'. Cara then gave us all an example. For her, something 'natural' is something that is self-evident. For Cara, however, something that is 'random' is something that is out of place: it is like a line up of objects equally spaced, and one is unequally spaced. For Cara, being a girl was all she had ever known. To have to deny that reality and be a boy solely on the basis of other people's expectations based on her genitalia would thus make her out of place.
>
> Hearing this, Amanda and Peter were able to acknowledge that since she could speak Cara had insisted that she was a girl, but that at first they had thought she just misunderstood pronouns. On reflection, however, they could see that Cara had never misgendered anyone else, and thus it was entirely reasonable that her description of her gender was entirely correct.

If we want to think about a general rule, we might suggest that an infant has a range of groupings that we as adults would see as pertaining to gender. For example, an infant might have one category that includes a diverse group of people who smell a particular way, who have a particular quality of voice, who touch with a particular degree of firmness, most of whom have shorter hair, and some of whom have facial hair. When the infant begins to acquire language, they notice that the people in this group are uniformly, or close to uniformly, referred to as 'he'. 'He' then becomes a linguistic descriptor through which to label this group. Might there have been some people who are not 'he', but who previously fell into this group? Almost certainly. There will have been women with facial hair, and some men with long hair. But the limitations of language will draw tighter boundaries around this group, limiting it to people who are referred to as 'he'.

The million dollar question with regard to gender, however, goes beyond how infants categorise people, and then how the categories they develop become attached to a limited linguistic structure that translates grey into black and white. The real question at the heart of the matter, as signalled by the questions that parents ask me, is how we *know* our gender. Importantly in this regard, Fausto-Sterling (2012) suggests that gender is about affinities. Importantly, the point that Fausto-Sterling makes it not about some sort of automaticity that translates affect to identity. Further, it is not about affinity with a particular person (so it is not *per se* about affinity with the gender of a parent). Rather, it is about an affinity that arises from the sensory inputs that are collected into category groupings that later become known as gender. Importantly, this might require a compromise. It might be that, prior to language, a child has a diverse number of categories that through language must be translated into a gender category that describes their own affinity with a particular category. The actual pre-linguistic category that an infant feels affinity with might not be entirely represented by one of the binary genders of male and female made available to them, so most (though not all) children will make a compromise about which of the two most commonly available gender categories best represents their own cognitive categories, and specifically the one they feel an affinity with.

Gender, then, is what we feel. It is not about our genitalia, and it is not just about our tone of voice, or hair length, or the forms of play we prefer to engage in, or firmness of touch. It is about how, cumulatively, a range of sensory inputs make us feel, and whether those feelings that we experience when reduced through language to a binary system of categorisation are experienced as familiar and 'like' us, or whether they feel different to us. Again, importantly, there is likely considerable diversity in these categories of feeling prior to language, and most certainly more than two categories. As I noted above, whilst we know that most children end up feeling most at home within one of two binary gender categories (including children who are transgender), some children do not, and this speaks, I would suggest, to the capacity of some children to resist the limitations of gender categories within language, and to maintain within themselves a connection to the greyness of categorisation that likely existed prior to language.

Specifically in terms of transgender children who have a binary gender, prior to language they will have collected a range of sensory information into groupings, and as they enter into language and also become able to see themselves as distinct entities, they will experience themselves as having an affinity with one binary category over the other. It is understandable, then, that when such children hear pronouns used that describe one category that is not their own, and when those same pronouns are used to describe them, there will be some form of cognitive dissonance.

In terms of gender diversity more broadly, some children might reconcile any sense of cognitive dissonance by expanding the category that is being applied to them so that it encompasses their own feelings. This might speak to the experiences of a diverse range of children who are in some way gender non-conforming (such as children who are assigned male, who engage in play and behaviours that are not stereotypically male, but who are comfortable to differing degrees with the category 'male'). Other children might do their very best to cognitively avoid associating their experiences of self with the labels applied to them by others. This might speak to the experiences of children who disclose that they are transgender in late childhood or in the teenage years, at a point where strategies of avoidance become untenable. Finally, there will be other children who from a young age externalise the dissonance, pointing out to others that they are mistaken in their attributions. These are the very young children who, from the time they can speak, assert their gender and in some cases are affirmed by their parents. Importantly, cross cutting these three categories (and there may be many other categories) is a central focus on comfort and affinity. Transgender children who assert their gender should not be approached by clinicians in a way that attempts to paint them simply as 'gender non-conforming'. The very basic typology I outline above both recognises a degree of overlap between the categories, but also is very clear that each evokes different levels of comfort and affinity, and this is what should guide clinicians, not a desire to assert gender non-conformity in the face of a child who clearly has voiced a gender denoting that they are transgender.

As I have argued in this section, what we think of as gender is first a process of categorisation that is grey, diverse, and based on affect. As a child enters into language and comes to see themselves as an individual entity, they may be confronted with a discrepancy between the category they have allocated to themselves based on affinity, and the category others have them placed in. The evidence on early understandings of what is thought of as gender has too often assumed that this in fact references sex. As I have argued above, this is a fallacy, and that instead what very young children are doing is creating groupings so as to order their world, groupings that typically have very little to do with visual inspection of the genitalia of others. That transgender children make such groupings is entirely unsurprising, just as is it entirely unsurprising that transgender children with a binary gender would experience an affinity with one particular category, and engage in a range of strategies to expand, avoid, or correct the incorrect assumptions made about the category they experience an affinity with. In the box below I consider the second aspect of the GENDER case formulation, focusing on how despite Cara's clear description of her gender, her parents still expressed concerns.

Case Study 1: Expressed Concerns

In our second session, Amanda and Peter returned to their earlier questions about how they can be 'sure' about Cara's gender. In order to unpack this with them, I worked through some of the concepts that I explored in the section above. Specifically, I asked Amanda and Peter to unpack their own understandings of their gender. Amanda shared that when she was young people called her a 'tomboy', because she liked to have short hair and enjoyed playing football. Amanda said that she never had anyone question that she was a girl, but that being called a tomboy had at times been distressing for her, and she perceived it as a derogatory term. I asked Amanda to elaborate how she knew, in the face of not conforming to social stereotypes about 'appropriate' behaviours for girls, that she knew she was in fact a girl, Amanda stated, just like Cara, that it was something she had known as long as she could remember, and that it felt 'natural' when people referred to her as 'she'.

Turning to speak with Peter, he shared that he had grown up in a strict religious household, which offered no space to think critically about gender. In his family children born with a penis were boys and were expected to look and act in a certain way, and children born with a vagina were girls and were also expected to look and act in a particular way. On reflection Peter could see that the roles accorded to his family members, and particularly to his mother, were often oppressive, and left no space to explore a diversity of interests and expressions. Peter acknowledged that he didn't want to be like his own father, and shut down Cara's gender expression. More broadly, he also acknowledged that he wanted his children to be accepting of other people, and to feel free to explore the world on their own terms. Indeed, he had distanced himself from his family in order to get away from the religion that he found oppressive growing up, but was mindful that sometimes he slipped back into the black and white thinking that had shaped his childhood.

Listening to all of this, Cara was clearly moved by her parents' childhood experiences, having previously heard little about them. Cara was able to draw parallels between her own experiences in relation to gender and her parents' experiences. Without explicitly referencing cisgenderism, Cara spoke about how all three of them had felt shut down by other people's expectations, and she was excited by the idea that her parents were showing greater understanding of her gender, and seemed more willing to be affirming.

Cisgenderism in Theories of Gendered Understandings

In the previous section I elaborated an account of how young children come to view themselves as inhabiting a particular gender, and how this builds on pre-verbal categorisations that children develop when attempting to cognitively organise the world around them. In this section I draw on three particular strands of research to outline in further detail how gender as a category becomes salient to children, and how this research has often relied upon cisgenderist assumptions, and how this operates to marginalise transgender children. Building on the previous section, however, I also demonstrate that existing approaches can be reframed through an affirming lens so as to be inclusive of transgender children.

Social Learning Approach

The first of the three strands adopts a social learning approach to children's understandings of gender. Social learning approaches in general emphasise modelling as the key way in which children learn social rules and categories. With regard to gender, social learning theorists, starting with the early work of Mischel (1966), suggest that a child who is positively reinforced for engaging in particular gender stereotyped behaviours comes to accept that the gender to which the stereotypes relate is their own. There are, however, a number of problems associated with this account. First, and as Bem (1983) argued, social learning theory sees children as passive recipients of the world around them. As I argued in the previous section, children are far from passive recipients, even if their cognitive appraisals of the world around them may at times be limited by the language available to them. Second, and with specific focus on transgender children, assumptions about the nexus between reinforcement and gender is particularly vexed. A child who engages in particular gender stereotyped behaviours may not be rewarded if the adults who surround them believe that the behaviours are not appropriate. For example, a child assigned male at birth who enjoys playing with toys stereotypically given to girls, and who has located themselves in the category 'female' may not be encouraged or rewarded for doing so. The same child may nonetheless strongly assert their gender as female, despite a lack of external reinforcement.

Socio-cognitive Approach

The second strand of research that focuses on how children learn about gender adopts a social-cognitive approach. Different to social learning – which emphasises the idea that behaviours lead to understanding – social-cognitive approaches suggest the opposite: that understanding leads to behaviours. Drawing on the early work of Kohlberg (1966), social-cognitive approaches suggest that children must first learn to self-categorise with regard to gender, and to be able to categorise the gender of others. Early research suggested that children do not demonstrate the ability to categorise until on average six years of age, but subsequent research has suggested that this may occur much earlier, between two and three years of age (Bussey and Bandura 1999). Second, children must come to understand that gender is constant: that it does not change over time. Research suggests that this occurs on average in the fifth year of a child's life (Ruble et al. 2007). And finally, children come to appreciate that despite any physical changes in a person's appearance (i.e., longer hair or shorter hair), their gender remains the same.

I would argue here that of the three approaches to be outlined in this section, social-cognitive approaches are the most clearly cisgenderist in their theorising of gender development. Social-cognitive approaches are cisgenderist in the way that they presume that in first learning to self-categorise their gender, a child's gender should normatively reflect their assigned sex. So a child who was assigned female at birth but who states that their gender is male is viewed within a social-cognitive approach as having failed to achieve a basic understanding of gender. This is most starkly evident in a study of transgender children, which sought to assess gender constancy judgments (Zucker et al. 1999). The study concluded that the transgender children in the study displayed a 'developmental lag' in understanding gender, because they could not 'correctly' identify their gender at the same age as their cisgender peers. 'Correctly', however, referred to children accepting the cisgenderist assumption that their assigned sex determined their gender. It is no surprise that young transgender children who were clear about their gender asserted this, and that it took several years for them to 'accept' the social norms imposed on them.

Examples of the cisgenderism inherent to social-cognitive theories of gender are also evident in the measures used to assess children's understandings of gender. These include asking children to 'match' figures normatively marked as male or female (via clothing, hair, etc) with particular roles or objects. Thinking back to the previous section, these types of tests do not involve the child knowing anything about the genitalia of the figures they are shown. Yet researchers make the assumption that because young children have learnt how to categorise people using available stereotypes and linguistic descriptors, that the attributions they make relate to assigned sex, rather than social norms about gender categories. To rewrite social-cognitive theories, then, we may suggest that first children come to categorise others (as outlined in the previous section of this chapter), and then come to categorise themselves (again as outlined in the previous section). With these processes of categorisation in place and their association with available linguistic categories, children are then able to more finely tune the categories they have developed. This tuning occurs in the context of multiple sources of inputs that repeatedly assert a limited range of stereotypes about each of two binary genders, through which children will learn which behaviours are taboo for each gender. As such, it is perhaps less that children learn that gender *does not* change, but rather they learn, in a context of cisgenderism, that gender is seen as immutable, and that it is determined by assigned sex. This point about assigned sex is evident in the assumption within social-cognitive approaches that children learn that cosmetic changes do not alter gender. In reality, this assumption reflects the idea that there is an immutable basis to gender, namely genitalia.

Recent research with transgender children affirms the account I have provided above in my reworking of social-cognitive approaches. Yes, from a very young age transgender children categorise others, and when they learn to speak they learn to attach these categorisations to available linguistic categories. Transgender children at this point will already know their gender, though will also come to know that other people misapprehend their gender. Nonetheless, they will continue (even if, for some children, facing considerable prohibition) to engage in behaviours and interests that align with their gender. In so doing, they display an awareness that their gender does not change, but likely also an awareness that their gender falls outside the spectrum of what other people expect of them based on their genitalia. Knowing about this disjuncture between other people's expectations and their own experiences, transgender children become finely attuned to appreciating that gender is not determined by genitalia but rather by affinity and feeling. As such, it is unsurprising that research has found that when we focus on gender rather than assigned sex, transgender children understand gender as a category and their own gender at the same age as do cisgender children, that they know that their gender will not change, but they nonetheless appreciate that changes in physical appearance *can* reflect a change in a person's gender (Fast and Olson 2018). This says nothing about a 'developmental lag' in transgender children, and everything about their capacity to resist the normative association between assigned sex and gender, and to be affirming of other people with regard to gender. In the box below I explore the third aspect of the GENDER case formulation with regard to Cara in terms of the necessary actions that arose when her parents became more affirming of her gender.

> **Case Study 1: Necessary Actions**
> In our third session, Cara presented with a very clear agenda to negotiate her social transition at school. Cara spoke about again feeling very 'random' that at home she wears her clothes borrowed from her sister, but at school she has to wear her old clothes. Cara also spoke about being grateful that at home most of the time her parents and siblings call her by her name, and use the correct pronouns, but that at school this doesn't happen, and it was becoming increasingly distressing. Amanda and Peter could see that not progressing social transition at school was holding Cara back, and that they needed to take action sooner rather than later.
> Amanda and Peter stated that, following the previous session, they felt much more confident that not only did they understand the importance of affirming Cara, but that they felt more suitably equipped to convince others of this, including the school. We spoke about some of the research that

I outlined in the section above about gender awareness and children's development, and Amanda and Peter noted that they felt this was really important information for them to have so that they could clearly advocate to the school, which they feared would be not entirely supportive given Cara's age.

In order to try and increase the likelihood that the school would be supportive, I worked with Amanda and Peter to identify the relevant government policies that they could draw upon to advocate for Cara, and also linked them in with a local programme that provides education to schools and advocates for the inclusion of transgender children. Amanda and Peter noted that they had already shared information about Cara with some close and trusted parents at the school, who had offered to come on board as additional support should the school prove to be less than supportive. With Cara, we discussed a realistic time frame within which Amanda and Peter would approach the school, discuss Cara's requirements (such as using the girls' toilets), and the point and manner in which Cara's class would be informed.

Gender Schema Theory

The third strand of research was developed by Bem (1983), and is known as gender schema theory. A schema is an ideological system that attributes particular meaning to a given phenomenon, translating something absent of inherent meaning (i.e., in regards to gender; genitalia), into a complex web of normative meanings and stereotypes. To a certain degree, gender schema theory is also mired in cisgenderism, in that it assumes that children first come to know the 'truth' of their assigned sex, and then come to learn the schema about gender that frames who they can or cannot be, on the basis of their assigned sex. Bem is right in suggesting that this acknowledges that children learn a set of rules that they can resist or conform to, but it is fundamentally flawed in the assumption that children will resist or conform on the basis of knowledge about their assigned sex, rather on the basis of their gender. This is most evident where Bem speaks about how to raise children able to resist dominant gender schemas. Bem suggests that she taught her children to know that yes, your genitalia determine what you are, but they do not determine what you can do. Bem's intention was to challenge gender stereotypes, but unfortunately in so doing she reified assigned sex as the determinant of gender.

Research undertaken since Bem (1983) elaborated her account of gender schema theory suggests that grounding schemas on children's presumed awareness of assigned sex and acceptance that assigned sex determines gender may well be unfounded. For example, researchers have found that some young children believe that genitalia can change with time (Frey and Ruble 1992), and that genitalia may not be viewed by some children as bearing any relationship to particular gendered interests or behaviours. That these findings are often overlooked or minimised speaks to an investment on the part of researchers in maintaining the belief that assigned sex determines gender, and that 'correct' understandings are based on both the internalisation of cisgenderism, and the internalisation of 'appropriate' gendered behaviours and interests. As we shall see in the following section, this type of investment has implications for the diagnostic tools used by clinicians who work with transgender children.

Cisgenderism, Developmentalism and Transgender Children

Before turning to consider how cisgenderism shapes diagnostic tools used by clinicians when working with transgender children, it is important to first state strongly and clearly that such diagnostic tools are not necessary, and in many national contexts are not mandatory. Certainly in some national contexts, a formal diagnosis may be necessary in order for health insurance to be used, but in many other contexts a formal diagnosis is not required in order to support and affirm transgender child in the clinical setting. Even in contexts where a diagnosis is required, as clinicians we must be very careful not to treat diagnoses as central to the work that we do with transgender children. Rather, if a diagnosis is required by health insurers then this can be undertaken simply and directly for that purpose, quite separate from the work that we do to affirm and support transgender children. Indeed, instead of sitting down with a child and working systematically through the diagnostic criteria, we can instead draw on our broader conversations with children to identify whether a diagnosis might be warranted.

With the above points in mind about when we might or might not use diagnostic tools, and how if we do use them we must do so in respectful and affirming ways, we can now turn to consider how past and current diagnostic tools are both cisgenderist, and also developmentalist. Developmentalism refers to normative assumptions often inherent to developmental psychology, where various stage models claim to account for how the 'average' child will (or indeed should) develop, thus providing a means by which to identify children whose development is 'atypical' (Burman 1994; Walkerdine 1993). Further, developmentalism suggests that adults are those best placed to know how children should develop, to monitor their development, and to intervene when something is perceived as 'wrong' with a child's development. Certainly we could view claims about transgender children displaying a 'developmental lag' as both a form of cisgenderism and a form of developmentalism.

Turning to consider the American Psychiatric Association's *Diagnostic and Statistical Manual of Mental Disorders* (DSM), it is useful to begin by looking at the fourth edition (2000), which included the diagnosis of 'gender identity disorder'. This diagnosis provided two different categories: one for children, and one for adolescents and adults. Importantly, I would note here that in its discussion of 'gender identity disorder', the fourth edition of the DSM provides no discussion of the formation of gender as a general category, instead treating gender as an automatic correlate of assigned sex, and hence treating transgender people as a problem in need of explanation. An example of this appears in the diagnostic criteria for children included in the fourth edition, which discuss the 'failure' of transgender children to develop friendships and interests appropriate to their age. Here the fourth edition diagnosis of 'gender identity diagnosis' accepts the assumption that age appropriate friendships and interests should be normatively gendered, such that children assigned male should play with other children assigned male and should engage in activities stereotypically associated with male assigned children, and vice versa for children assigned female. This type of assumption is not only cisgenderist, but it is also developmentalist in that it treats divergence from a norm as a 'failure'.

The fifth edition of the DSM purportedly sought to address what were seen as pathologising aspects of the diagnosis of 'gender identity disorder', specifically by reframing the diagnosis as 'gender dysphoria' (American Psychiatric Association 2013). The key difference in the two diagnoses is that whilst in the fourth edition 'gender identity disorder' referred to the general fact of being transgender, 'gender dysphoria' refers primarily to distress related to being transgender, specifically with regard to one's body. Yet despite this shift in nomenclature, much of the diagnosis of 'gender dysphoria' reads like the previous diagnosis of 'gender identity disorder'. Again, the development of gender is not discussed in any detail, and whilst the introduction to the diagnostic criteria goes to some lengths to distinguish sex from gender, it ends up implicitly collapsing the two by referring to 'natal gender', which is assigned at birth. The suggestion that gender is assigned at birth defaults to genitalia as the key determining factor in 'natal gender', as evident in the statement that "in contrast to certain social constructionist theories, biological factors are seen as contributing [to gender], in interaction with social and psychological factors" (p. 451).

Further, the fifth edition diagnosis of 'gender dysphoria', specifically with regard to children, includes the repeated use of the word 'incongruence'. Here we can see the cisgenderist assumption that there should be some 'congruence' between assigned sex and gender. As I explored in detail in the previous two sections, assigned sex is primarily based on visual inspection of the genitalia. Gender, by contrast, is an entirely different phenomenon, based on one's subjective experience of the world around us, and of our relationship to it. In other words, it is something that can only be known and described once we ourselves are able to do so: it cannot be assigned by another person. Admittedly, there is some form of 'congruence' between assigned sex and gender for the vast majority of the population, but this, I would argue, is something of a red herring. It is a red herring because the emphasis on 'congruence' treats something that is true for a majority of people as true for all people, and it also treats this truth as an acontextual and ahistorical fact. It is well documented that the attachment of something called 'gender' to genitalia is a relatively recent phenomenon amongst humans (Scott 1986).

Further examples of cisgenderism appear in the fifth edition of the DSM in repeated references to 'cross-gender identification'. Here we must ask 'across from what'? If, as I carefully elaborated in the previous sections of this chapter, children have an understanding of their gender from a very young age, and if this bears no inherent relationship to their assigned sex, then a child's 'gender identifications' are simply that when it comes to transgender children: they are the same as any child's gender identifications that are based on feelings and affinity, rather than on a normative relationship to assigned sex. Cisgenderism is also evident in the diagnosis of 'gender dysphoria' when the case for the specific diagnostic criterion is based upon recourse to "well documented behavioural gender differences between typically developing boys and girls" (p. 455). This statement not only frames transgender children as atypical, but it also insists that 'well documented behavioural gender differences' should not equally apply to transgender children as they do to cisgender children. The reason why they do not apply, according to the implicit assumption of the DSM, is that gender is determined by assigned sex.

Finally in terms of the DSM diagnosis of 'gender dysphoria', reference is made to a difference between 'early' as compared to 'late' onset gender dysphoria. The former refers to young children who disclose that they are transgender, whilst the latter refers to disclosures made during the teenage years. This distinction, I would argue, is a form of developmentalism, in that it both potentially implies that a young transgender child who knows and asserts their gender is 'too young' to know, and conversely that older children who assert their gender are delayed in their awareness of their gender. This argument as included in the fifth edition of the DSM is a form of eating one's cake and having it too, driven, it would seem, by a set of underlying assumptions about what children can and cannot know, and the degree to which adults should put faith in transgender children's accounts of their gender. This point is particularly vexed with regard to a pseudo 'diagnosis' that increasingly circulates in some circles that are not affirming of transgender children, namely 'rapid onset gender dysphoria'. Framed as a diagnosis, 'rapid onset gender dysphoria' is actually a concept used to deny the legitimacy of transgender children's gender (see Jones 2017; Serano 2018 for a discussion). The suggestion inherent to the concept is that children 'suddenly' disclose that they are transgender, with no documented history of the gender that they disclose. The argument made by proponents of the concept is that children are 'coached' to believe that they are transgender by peers. Whilst the concept of 'rapid onset gender dysphoria' is in no way endorsed by the DSM, I would suggest that discussions about 'onset' included in the fifth edition have unintentionally paved the way for 'onset' to be seen as a valid diagnostic consideration, one laden with cisgenderist and developmentalist assumptions.

In the box below I consider the fourth aspect of the GENDER case formulation, specifically with regard to the school's response to Cara and the distress this produced.

Case Study 1: Distress Management

A period of time passed before our next appointment, during which Amanda and Peter had planned to approach the school and negotiate a realistic time frame for Cara's social transition. Ahead of the appointment Amanda made contact to let me know that the school was being less than supportive, and that this was making Cara distressed, to the point that she was acting out both in class and at home. I offered to Amanda that I could meet with the school to discuss their concerns, which Amanda agreed would be helpful.

When I met with the school principal and counsellor, they began by acknowledging that they are absolutely in support of transgender people, but that they felt that at age eight some caution should be applied with regard to Cara. They also felt that, given they had not seen any 'signs' at school, that it seemed very sudden to announce that Cara was in fact a girl. At this point I asked if the class teacher could join us, and luckily she was available. When I asked the class teacher about 'signs', she acknowledged that Cara only had female friends, and that there had been moments when Cara had shown intense discomfort using the boy's toilet and lining up with boys. The principal asked if this was simply immaturity on Cara's part, and that perhaps the school could 'help' by pairing Cara up with a male buddy in class so that she could make friends with boys.

At this point I asked all three staff members what they thought a school could expect of an eight year old student in terms of maturity. They outlined their expectations re: behaviour, following rules, understanding authority, and showing consideration to other students. I reflected to them that these are all significant expectations of relatively young students in terms of maturity, and asked if they felt that Cara in general succeeded in meeting these expectations. All could acknowledge that Cara was indeed very mature for her age, which afforded me the space to ask why, then, we would expect that Cara was too young to know her gender. This gave all three pause for thought, and led to them acknowledging that some of their responses were driven by fear about how other families in the school might react to Cara, and that they had also read information online about transgender children that, it would seem, was misinformation about gender and development.

I agreed that I would share further information with the school to aid in their learning, and the principal reported that he was more than happy to meet with the parents again to negotiate a time frame for Cara's social transition. When I then met with Cara, Amanda, and Peter, Cara still reported feeling distress about how the school had responded, but felt increasingly positive that the social transition was on the near horizon, and that her class teacher in particular seemed very understanding and supportive.

Shifting from the DSM, I now turn to consider the World Professional Association for Transgender Health's *Standards of Care* (SOC), now in their seventh edition (2011). The SOC, as compared to the DSM, are widely seen as more affirming in their approach to working with transgender people in a clinical context, and certainly as less pathologising. Indeed, the SOC make a clear distinction between dysphoria and pathology, recognise a diversity of genders, and do not emphasise the need for a formal diagnosis. Yet even with these positive aspects of the SOC in mind, a paper by Castañeda (2015) makes a cogent argument for the developmentalism inherent to the SOC. Castañeda points towards the distinction made in the SOC between children and adolescents as functioning to treat the former as experiencing considerable 'fluidity and variability', and with the latter marked as moving towards a state of fixity. The assumption that normative development is marked by a move from fluidity to fixity, Castañeda suggests, enables the SOC to include a discussion of the problematic concepts of 'persistence' and 'desistence'. Derived from earlier research that has now been shown to be problematic (Temple Newhook et al. 2018), these concepts place under question transgender children's gender, suggesting that many children who report that they are transgender may grow up to be otherwise. The distinction made between fluidity and fixity in the SOC thus allows for caution to be applied when working with young children, when in reality and as this book argues, such caution is not warranted, and certainly is not a feature of an affirming approach. In the box below I explore the fourth strand of the GENDER case formulation, focusing on how, when we shift away from thinking about fluidity and fixity of key markers of whether or not to affirm transgender children, this opens us up to a broad range of opportunities.

Case Study 1: Ecologies of Support

At our next session, Amanda and Peter reported that whilst changes at school had been happening gradually (and for Cara a little too gradually), they were pleased with the support they had eventually received, and that it appeared that the school community were in general being supportive. They wondered, however, about what else they could do to encourage support and understanding for their family. Amanda and Peter shared that they were well known within the school community, and felt that they wanted a way to reach out to people who may be struggling, or who may be greater allies than Amanda and Peter perhaps knew.

One suggestion I offered to the family was to throw a party celebrating Cara, so that everyone had the opportunity to see the family as a united front, and also for Cara to feel affirmed by all. The parents felt that this was a great idea, and had similarly heard of parents placing 'birth' notices in the paper to celebrate a child's gender. We agreed that inviting the entire school would be unmanageable, so we focused on identifying people who were already great supports for the family and who could be relied upon at the party, but also people whom the family had long-standing relationships with, but whom appeared to be taking extra time to be affirming of Cara.

Together we came up with the idea of sending out two different invitations. To the people who were already supportive (and this included extended family members), the invitation was simply to a party to celebrate Cara. To the people who Amanda and Peter believed were struggling, the invitation was to a 'space of learning', and was accompanied with some basic information they had collected about transgender children, and which had been a great help to them. Amanda and Peter thus saw the party as both an opportunity to celebrate and an opportunity to educate.

Following the party Amanda contacted me to let me know that it had been a great success. Only one person had come up to her and let her know that despite the information and their acknowledgement that all they wanted was for Cara to be happy, they still had some concerns and would need 'more time to think'. But this person aside, Amanda was heartened by the fact that some people whom before had been struggling, now seemed to be strong allies to the family.

Castañeda (2015) also critiques the argument provided in the SOC that differing treatments for transgender children are also premised upon assumptions about fluidity and fixity. Specifically, Castañeda suggests that puberty blockers for transgender children are framed as fully reversible, whilst hormone therapy for older adolescents are framed as only partially reversible. This distinction, Castañeda suggests, is developmentalist, in that it repeats the assumption that young children don't truly know their gender, and that only when we can be certain that they do would we endorse treatments that are only partially reversible. The problem with this logic is that we don't equally apply it to most cisgender children (though see Pyne 2017 for a notable exception, and additional discussion about transgender children and temporality). We don't prescribe puberty blockers for cisgender children so that they can move towards a greater state of 'fixity' in their gender before they are capable of experiencing puberty. Yet for transgender children we 'suppress' puberty – often referred to as 'hitting the pause button' – so that enough time can pass that children are more developmentally able to be sure about their gender and any treatments they may undertake. Again, we don't do this with cisgender children, so what we are in fact doing is treating transgender children as incapable of knowing their gender with any certainty, a form of both cisgenderism and developmentalism. Given what we know of the distress that many transgender adolescents experience in regards to not going through puberty along with their peers (Strauss et al. 2017), the logic inherent to the SOC may be seen as less than affirming.

Concluding Thoughts

From her research with young transgender people, Singh (2013) reports that many of the young people she spoke with viewed developmentalism as a key barrier to receiving support. Specifically, her participants stated that parents, school staff, and healthcare professionals all gave the message that young transgender people need to 'wait and see', based on the assumption that young people do not fully understand their gender. For Singh's participants this meant that whilst some of the adults in their networks were in general affirming, in the specific (i.e., in terms of commencing hormone therapy) they often declined to be supportive, under the rhetoric of 'waiting and seeing', based on developmentalist assumptions about when the beliefs and experiences of children can be trusted. As I will explore in the final aspect of the GENDER case formulation in the box below, however, it is important that in seeking to avoid developmentalist assumptions about transgender children, we do not eschew the important affirming role we can play as adults equipped with considerable epistemic authority, though we should always do so mindful of the resistances that children make in the face of a lack of support.

> **Case Study 1: Reinforcement and Resistance**
>
> Throughout this case study there have, of course, been examples of reinforcement that I provided to the family. Sometimes this involved reinforcing best practice evidence from a critical perspective, and other times it involved giving the parents permission to work through their own beliefs and challenges, so that they could become advocates for their daughter. Reinforcement can also involve going out into the community to be an advocate, such as going into the school to speak with staff.
>
> In terms of resistance, I like to think of Cara's framing of 'natural' and 'random' as a point of resistance. Certainly, Cara could speak clearly and eloquently about her gender, this was never in doubt. But that she could frame her account in a way that resisted the cisgenderist assumption that genitalia determines gender and in so doing claiming the category 'natural' for herself was, I think, particularly insightful. This is not to say that Cara did not have to contend with multiple adults struggling to understand her, and that this had a very real impact upon her. Rather, it is to acknowledge resistance in the face of a relative lack of support and understanding.

In conclusion, in this chapter I have gone into considerable detail about how exactly we can be sure about a child's gender, and how we can have confidence that a child knows their gender. Certainly it will remain the case that some parents will struggle to accept that their child knows that of which they speak. Cisgenderism and developmentalism are prevalent ideologies in most national contexts, and they fundamentally shape whether or not we will view children as experts on any topic, let alone their gender. Working through what we know from the research about gender development, as was evident in the case study presented in this chapter, offers one way of helping parents move from a space of uncertainty, to a space of affirmation. This requires us as clinicians to be able to carefully unpack the assumptions that many parents bring with them, assumptions that, as we have explored in this chapter, are reinforced in the much of the literature. As I elaborated in Chap. 1, as scientist-practitioners we must bring a critical developmental lens to bear upon cisgenderist assumptions, so that the knowledge we share with the parents we work with is affirming of transgender children.

References

American Psychiatric Association. (2000). *DSM-IV-TR: Diagnostic and statistical manual of mental disorders*. Washington, DC: American Psychiatric Association.

American Psychiatric Association. (2013). *Diagnostic and statistical manual of mental disorders (DSM-5)*. Washington, DC: American Psychiatric Association.

Bem, S. L. (1983). Gender schema theory and its implications for child development: Raising gender-aschematic children in a gender-schematic society. *Signs: Journal of Women in Culture and Society, 8*(4), 598–616.

Burman, E. (1994). *Deconstructing developmental psychology*. London: Routledge.

Bussey, K., & Bandura, A. (1999). Social cognitive theory of gender development and differentiation. *Psychological Review, 106*(4), 676.

Castañeda, C. (2015). Developing gender: The medical treatment of transgender young people. *Social Science & Medicine, 143*, 262–270.

Fast, A. A., & Olson, K. R. (2018). Gender development in transgender preschool children. *Child Development, 89*(2), 620–637.

Fausto-Sterling, A. (2012). The dynamic development of gender variability. *Journal of Homosexuality, 59*(3), 398–421.

Frey, K. S., & Ruble, D. N. (1992). Gender constancy and the 'cost' of sex-typed behavior: A test of the conflict hypothesis. *Developmental Psychology, 28*(4), 714–721.

Jones, Z. (2017). *Fresh trans myth of 2017: 'Rapid onset gender dysphoria'*. Retrieved August 31, 2018, from https://genderanalysis.net/2017/07/fresh-trans-myths-of-2017-rapid-onset-gender-dysphoria/

Kohlberg, L. (1966). A cognitive-developmental analysis of children's sex-role concepts and attitudes. In E. E. Maccoby (Ed.), *The development of sex differences* (pp. 82–173). Stanford: Stanford University Press.

Martin, C. L., Ruble, D. N., & Szkrybalo, J. (2002). Cognitive theories of early gender development. *Psychological Bulletin, 128*(6), 903.

Mischel, W. (1966). A social-learning view of sex differences in behavior. In E. E. Maccoby (Ed.), *The development of sex differences* (pp. 57–81). Stanford: Stanford University Press.

Owen Blakemore, J. E., Berenbaum, S. A., & Liben, L. S. (2009). *Gender development*. New York: Psychology Press.

Pyne, J. (2017). Arresting Ashley X: Trans youth, puberty blockers and the question of whether time is on your side. *Somatechnics, 7*(1), 95–123.

Ruble, D. N., Taylor, L. J., Cyphers, L., Greulich, F. K., Lurye, L. E., & Shrout, P. E. (2007). The role of gender constancy in early gender development. *Child Development, 78*(4), 1121–1136.

Scott, J. W. (1986). Gender: A useful category of historical analysis. *The American Historical Review, 91*(5), 1053–1075.

Serano, J. (2018, August 22). Everything you need to know about rapid onset gender dysphoria. *Medium*. Retrieved August 31, 2018, from https://medium.com/@juliaserano/everything-you-need-to-know-about-rapid-onset-gender-dysphoria-1940b8afdeba

Singh, A. A. (2013). Transgender youth of color and resilience: Negotiating oppression and finding support. *Sex Roles, 68*(11–12), 690–702.

Strauss, P., Cook, A., Winter, S., Watson, V., Wright Toussaint, D., & Lin, A. (2017). *Trans pathways: The mental health experiences and care pathways of trans young people*. Telethon Kids Institute, Perth.

Temple Newhook, J., Pyne, J., Winters, K., Feder, S., Holmes, C., Tosh, J., Sinnott, M.-L., Jamieson, A., & Pickett, S. (2018). A critical commentary on follow-up studies and 'desistance' theories about transgender and gender-nonconforming children. *International Journal of Transgenderism, 19*(2), 212–224.

Walkerdine, V. (1993). Beyond developmentalism? *Theory & Psychology, 3*(4), 451–469.

World Professional Association for Transgender Health (WPATH). (2011). *Standards of care for the health of transsexual, transgender, and gender nonconforming people, 7th version*.

Zucker, K. J., Bradley, S. J., Kuksis, M., Pecore, K., Birkenfeld-Adams, A., Doering, R. W., Mitchell, J. N., & Wild, J. (1999). Gender constancy judgments in children with gender identity disorder: Evidence for a developmental lag. *Archives of Sexual Behavior, 28*(6), 475–502.

3

Challenges and Joys in Adolescence

For most adolescents, puberty is a time of considerable change that can bring with it both challenges and positive growth. Historically, much of the research on transgender adolescents has focused more on challenges, and very little on positive growth. In part this has been a product of clinical approaches that advocated for a 'wait and see' approach, as a result of which many transgender adolescents were forced to go through a puberty that was often intensely distressing. That such distress – accompanied by debates over whether making transgender adolescents go through the puberty normatively associated with their assigned sex was or was not ethical or best practice – has been the focus of the majority of research on transgender young people is hence not surprising. Yet as was outlined in the first chapter of this book, it is now widely accepted clinical practice that transgender young people should be supported to access puberty blockers and later to access hormones appropriate to their gender, if this is what they desire. In this context, puberty for transgender adolescents can look quite different to the experiences of distress widely documented in the literature. To date, however, a focus on distress remains a prevalent narrative in the literature, meaning that little space is devoted to exploring the positive growth that transgender young people may experience during adolescence.

This chapter seeks to address the limitations of past research on transgender adolescents by bringing together an account that focuses on both challenges and positive growth during adolescence for transgender young people. Importantly, focusing on growth is not intended to minimise challenges. Rather, the aim of this chapter is to provide something of an update or corrective to a literature that to date has primarily focused on the challenges. The young people I work with are most certainly attuned to the challenges that they face, and are often vocal in their opposition to the ways in which structural factors contribute to, or may be the source of, many of the challenges in their life (such as limited access to clinicians, long wait times, and legislative or clinical restrictions on their access to treatment). At the same time, however, the young people I work with respond creatively to the world around them, often experiencing adolescence as a time of significant growth and broadening of worldviews.

In order to map out both the challenges and positive growth that transgender adolescents experience, in this chapter I first consider how the developmental literature that has to date focused primarily on cisgender adolescents can speak to the experiences of transgender adolescents. In so doing I challenge the dominant framing of puberty as a biological process, instead looking at psychological maturation as a key component. This reframing allows for recognition of the fact that transgender adolescents who are currently prescribed puberty blockers are likely to experience many of the aspects of maturation experienced by their cisgender peers during puberty. At the same time, however, I critically examine the normative assumptions about gender inherent in much of the literature on adolescence and puberty. By locating such assumptions in a context of cisgenderism, I both highlight how this context produces many of the challenges that transgender young people face, and consider how transgender young people create spaces that resist particular normative developmental trajectories. Doing this allows for both an acknowledgement of the distress that some transgender young people experience in adolescence, and a consideration of the joys that they voice, and suggest that there are specific developmental tasks that clinicians can work on with transgender young people as part of adolescent growth.

Puberty as a Time of Intensification and Psychological Growth

In an early chapter on the topic of adolescence, Faust (1983) argued that in terms of child development, the categories we use are only made sense of within a particular way of thinking. More broadly, we know that 'adolescence' as a category is a relatively recent concept, one often used to regulate as much as it is purportedly used to liberate (Lesko 2012). Faust argued that not only do adults (including researchers and clinicians) impose particular ways of thinking on young people categorised as 'adolescents', but such young people both impose upon one another particular (normative) ways of thinking, and actively resist dominant ways of thinking so as to privilege their own worldviews. For transgender young people, it is thus vital that we situate them within the dominant ways of thinking likely elaborated by their peers and the adults in their lives, even if only to then consider how transgender adolescents may resist such dominant ways of thinking.

As was the case with the literature on gender development in childhood summarised in the previous chapter, the literature on adolescence is marked by a rigid gender binary, and moreover an emphasis upon gender that is treated as synonymous with assigned sex. As a result, much of the literature on adolescence emphasises what are seen as key differences between children assigned male or female. This is most evident in the ways in which the literature emphasises the effects of hormonal changes on the behaviours of children assigned female as compared to children assigned male. In this literature, puberty is a process through which children assigned male or female come into some sort of 'truth' about their gender that is assumed to be directly reflective of their assigned sex and the hormones associated with it. All of the stereotypes about female assigned children (other-oriented, thoughtful, emotionally expressive) and male assigned children (self-oriented, less focused on the needs of others, emotionally closed), within an understanding of puberty that emphasises hormones, are seen as direct reflections of a predetermined truth about gender rooted in biology. As we shall see in the second case study of the book below, these sorts of assumptions about puberty and hormones can have direct implications for young people.

> **Case Study 2: Gender Journey and Understanding**
>
> Jordan was fourteen when he first came to see me. At our first appointment Jordan told me that his parents, Ted and Julie, had been very reluctant to allow him to see me, and had only done so due to serious concerns about Jordan's self-harming. In our first appointment Jordan shared that he had asserted his gender as male from a very young age, but was met with constant rebuffs from his parents, who believed that young children often went through 'phases' and that Jordan would likely 'grow out of' the belief that he is male. For Jordan, this lack of support was an ongoing source of distress, and underpinned his self-harming.
>
> Also underpinning his self-harming was the fact that, due to the lack of support from his parents, Jordan had commenced puberty which did not fit with his gender, specifically beginning to menstruate and experiencing chest growth. Before this, Jordan had often been read by others outside his family as a boy, and this had brought him some happiness in the context of the lack of support at home. But the physical changes to his body wrought by puberty had meant that he was now rarely seen by others as a boy. Increased references to him as a girl were thus an additional cause of distress for Jordan, exacerbated by intense feelings of dysphoria brought on by puberty.

A different account of adolescence is provided by the concept of gender intensification (Hill and Lynch 1983). The gender intensification hypothesis argues that gender differences as they become more visible or salient during adolescence are a product of socialisation pressures that limit the ways in which young people are able to express themselves. For example, that girls may be more empathetic and caring than boys is not a product of assigned sex or a 'truth' about the nature of girls, but rather is a product of both what is expected of girls, and a rigid gender binary. To be intelligible as a girl requires conformity in some way to the stereotypes associated with girls. This is not to say that all girls will do this, but it is to say that there are considerable pressures to do so, and considerable prohibitions placed on girls who do not conform. The same can be said for boys. Importantly, however, gender intensification effects boys and girls differently, due to norms of masculinity and femininity. Hill and Lynch suggested that girls may have somewhat greater freedom to negotiate with normative expectations, whilst boys who undertake such negotiations may face higher levels of regulation (including physical violence), though of course this will differ depending on the context in which young people live, and it will likely also differ depending on whether the young person is cisgender or transgender.

Importantly, gender intensification during adolescence (i.e., a heightened focus on normative expectations about gender) comes from any number of sources. Parents may intentionally or unintentionally render gender norms salient. Consider, for example, the parent who asks a daughter if she wants children when she grows up, but does not ask a son the same question. This gives the message that particular things are expected of girls (or are expected to be central to their lives) that are not expected of boys in the same way. Peers are also a significant source of gender intensification. Peers may often regulate one another's actions or expressions, signalling what performances of gender are acceptable, which are relegated to the margins, and which are deemed unacceptable. As we shall see in the third case study below, for one young person the views of their peers played a significant role in shaping their understandings of gender. More widely, institutions such as the media give repeated messages about what is expected of young people based on their gender. That some young people resist normative messages in the context of gender intensification is thus something we should not lose sight of.

Case Study 3: Gender Journey and Understanding

Tania and her parents Bob and Francis first came to see me when Tania was seven. Bob and Francis had been extremely affirming and supportive of Tania from a very young age, and were seeking guidance on how best to support Tania into the future. One of the topics that we discussed was disclosure about Tania being transgender. Tania very much felt that it was information that did not need to be shared with people outside her family, or with anyone at school other than key members of staff directly involved with Tania. We spoke about the difference between a 'secret' and something that is 'private', and agreed that this information fell into the latter category. This framing helped Tania and her parents to see that whilst being secretive might lead to distress, viewing being transgender as a private matter was entirely reasonable.

I saw Tania and her parents infrequently for the following years, and was told that all was going well. Tania had many friends and enjoyed life. As puberty approached she was assessed for puberty blockers, and prescribed them at the appropriate age. Bob and Francis were staunch in their advocacy for Tania at school in terms of ensuring that teachers and other staff members maintained confidentiality about Tania's gender history, and this seemed to be working well. Tania reported being frustrated that she couldn't commence hormones until she was older, but was glad that she was not going through the puberty associated with her assigned sex.

For transgender young people specifically, the gender intensification hypothesis provides us with particular analytic leverage. Given the context of cisgenderism, and the assumption that gender is determined by assigned sex, gender intensification will be directed towards gender, even if it does not reflect assigned sex. As a result, transgender adolescents will typically experience the weight of gendered expectations not unlike that of their cisgender peers. However, in a way this is entirely different because the assumptions will relate to their assigned sex, not their gender. Many of the young people I work with speak of an intensification of gender approaching prior to and into the adolescent years, and for some this can result in acceding to the demand to conform, which often then leads to a 'break' where the young people discloses that they are transgender. Gender intensification, then, becomes a reason to disclose, so as to escape from normative gendered expectations that are distressing. As we will explore in the final section of this chapter, however, for some transgender young people this can mean stepping from one set of expectations into another, and this is something we can usefully explore in clinical work.

Case Study 2: Expressed Concerns

In a session with Ted and Julie alone, they sought to explain their lack of support for Jordan. Julie in particular noted that ahead of puberty, Jordan had grown his hair long, had started wearing nail polish, and had been working 'extra hard' to fit in with a group of female peers. For Ted and Julie this was evidence that Jordan was not transgender, but instead had 'just been going through a phase'. I emphasised to Ted and Julie that some young people do exactly this: in order to try to conform (often to avoid discrimination from peers), they will adopt styles of dress and mannerisms that closely mirror stereotypes associated with their assigned sex. This is not evidence of anything about their gender, but more about societal pressures to fit in. Ted and Julie acknowledged that this conformity only lasted for a short period of time, and seemed to only increase the distress that Jordan was experiencing, and indeed coincided with when Ted and Julie first became aware that Jordan was self-harming.

At a subsequent session I spoke to Jordan about past changes to his appearance. Jordan informed me that even though he knew that growing his hair long and wearing nail polish changed nothing about his gender, he felt that he needed to do something to make his parents happy, given they had expressed such unhappiness when he informed them that he was a boy. Unfortunately, if anything his attempts at conformity had only made Jordan more distressed, as they left him feeling that he didn't fit in anywhere: he didn't fit in with his family, he didn't fit in with female peers, he didn't fit in with male peers. Prior to his attempts at conformity Jordan had positive relationships with some of his male peers, however this had changed during his attempts at conformity, when his male friends had started treating him like a girl. When he cut his hair off again and returned to his previous masculine presentation, his male friends could not let go of their perception of him as female.

Further in terms of the gender intensification hypothesis, and different to biological accounts of puberty, for transgender young people adolescence can thus be a time of exploration. As I noted in the introduction to this chapter, this can often occur in absence of physical changes that are halted by the use of puberty blockers. Puberty blockers mean that transgender adolescents need not experience the physical aspects of a puberty associated with their assigned sex, but it does not mean that they do not grow. They come to understand processes of gender intensification, seeing what is expected of people on the basis of gender, and what this means for them. They must psychologically grapple with their cisgender peers experiencing the physical aspects of puberty, knowing that in most jurisdictions transgender young people do not have authorised access to hormones appropriate to their gender at similar ages. Yet despite this, they mature psychologically alongside their cisgender peers, coming to know themselves better, having skills for processing the expectations placed on them by the world around them, and fostering dreams for their future. As we shall explore in the following section, however, and different to their cisgender peers, transgender adolescents negotiate their lives in contexts that often cause distress.

Case Study 3: Expressed Concerns

When Tania turned 12, many of her female friends had already begun the physical changes associated with puberty, and Tania came to talk to me over a number of sessions about how she could manage the 'secret' and 'private' divide. Her friends had asked her if she had started menstruating, and whilst she didn't want to lie, she also didn't want to be an outsider. Francis had already offered to buy Tania a first bra, but Tania felt that wearing a bra would be lying, given she was not likely to experience any breast growth in the near future. Tania was also increasingly concerned about questions that might be asked of her with regards to changing rooms on school excursions, and why she changed clothes in a cubicle rather than out in the open along with her female peers.

For Tania, her perception of herself as an honest and caring person was fraught by her ongoing concerns about disclosure. Whilst she appreciated the distinction between a secret and something that is private, she nonetheless felt that being transgender was often akin to a secret, as it wasn't something she could speak about with her friends, and Tania experienced this as a barrier to close friendships. Tania wondered about whether some of her friends might be brought into a circle of trust, though both Bob and Francis were concerned that disclosure can't be undone, and they worried about whether other students at school could be trusted with the information.

Puberty as a Time of Discrimination and Distress

As I noted in the introduction to this chapter, the literature on transgender young people and adolescence has been dominated by a focus on distress. My goal in this chapter is to introduce additional foci to the study of adolescence for transgender young people, as we shall see in the following section. However, it is nonetheless important that as clinicians we are aware that despite an increasing shift towards an affirming model of care for transgender young people, a significant number of young people will still experience distress. In this section I explore two specific areas where distress can occur: in relation to one's body, and in regards to social relationships. It is important to emphasise again, as I do throughout this book, that cisgenderism plays a central role in producing much of the distress that transgender young people experience. Cisgenderism shapes how we see ourselves as much as it shapes how other people see us. As such, it is a powerful force regulating the lives of transgender young people.

Turning first to distress in relation to one's body, it is surprising to me that so much of the literature on 'dysphoria' as a category pertains almost solely to dysphoria as a diagnostic category. As I outlined in Chap. 2, the DSM5 (APA 2013) diagnosis of 'gender dysphoria' is limited by its cisgenderist and developmentalist framing. Also as I outlined in Chap. 2, using the DSM5 diagnosis as a primary lens through which to work with transgender young people inherently limits how we think about both gender and dysphoria. Certainly to a degree it makes sense that dysphoria in a diagnostic sense will predominate the literature, given that those advocating for an affirming approach to working with transgender children have had to fight against approaches that pathologise transgender people. This has certainly been of some success, with research demonstrating that as transgender people approach puberty they often experience considerable distress, which can be significantly reduced through the prescription of first puberty blockers and then hormones (De Vries et al. 2014). In the box below we take up the topic of puberty blockers with regards to the second case study. In this sense, dysphoria as diagnosis serves a function: it serves to warrant affirming treatments. Yet at the same time, a sole or primary focus on the diagnostic aspects of dysphoria does very little to encourage a focus on the phenomenology of dysphoria. Understanding what dysphoria actually *feels like* amongst young people for whom it is part of their lived experience is thus vital.

Case Study 2: Necessary Actions

As our sessions progressed, Ted and Julie slowly came to appreciate that their lack of support was causing Jordan considerable distress. Whilst they remained wedded to their view that gender is immutable and determined by assigned sex, they nonetheless wanted their child to be alive and happy. As a result, we discussed the possibility that Jordan might commence puberty blockers so as to cease his menstruation. This seemed to Jordan like a more viable option than starting the contraceptive pill, given such medication contains exactly the hormones that Jordan did not want in his body. Through our discussions Julie and Ted came to appreciate that puberty blockers are reversible, and that should they turn out to be 'right' and that this was 'just a phase', then Jordan would simply stop taking the blockers.

For Ted and Julie, then, the agreed upon necessary actions were not necessarily undertaken through a full appreciation of the effects of dysphoria, but rather were a product of their focus on Jordan's self-harming. Jordan and I spoke at length about his feelings of dysphoria, particularly with regard to menstruation as a signifier of femaleness, and how he was increasingly despondent about this. We also discussed in one-on-one sessions that Jordan doesn't need for blockers to be 'reversible' – he very clearly knows who he is. However we both were keenly aware of the narrative that his parents were wedded to, and that meeting his needs in terms of dysphoria unfortunately required some concessions in terms of how we presented information to his parents.

One key study that has focused on the lived experience of dysphoria (as opposed to dysphoria as a diagnostic category) involved a focus on body image amongst an international sample of 90 transgender young people aged between 15 and 26 years. From their interviews, McGuire, Doty, Catalpa and Ola (2016) report that their participants experienced both dissatisfaction and contentment with their bodies. In terms of the former, some of the participants described what McGuire and colleagues term 'disconnection' from particular aspects of their bodies that were experienced as misrepresentative of their gender (e.g., size of hands, or having a 'curvy' figure or not having a 'curvy' figure). For some participants, this disconnection served as a way to manage distress (i.e., by not thinking about particular body parts). Other participants who reported dissatisfaction focused on body size, with some using particular dietary regimes to alter their body size so that it better reflected their gender. Certainly the literature on adolescence more broadly emphasises a preoccupation amongst many adolescents with body size, however for transgender young people this takes particular forms as it intersects with gender self-representation. In other words, whilst, for example, girls in general may experience gender intensification as leading to particular concerns about body size, for transgender girls this may be exacerbated by where and how fat distributes, and how this is reflective or not of their gender according to social norms about how girls are expected to look.

In terms of contentedness, McGuire et al. (2016) report that for their participants who were able to access hormones, and for whom this resulted in physical changes, this bodily reshaping resulted in greater happiness and reduced feelings of dysphoria. Importantly, greater happiness did not simply reflect a more positive evaluation of their own bodies, but it also reflected that for some of the participants physical changes altered how they were viewed by others, often resulting in a reduction in misgendering, for example. Yet other participants who did not have access to hormones, or who did not see hormones as part of their journey, found other ways to narrate their bodies as sites of empowerment and pleasure, as we shall see in the following section of this chapter. This point is important, as it would be reductive to suggest that dysphoria can be totally ameliorated by the prescription of hormones.

Rather, it requires a shift both within the individual in terms of how they see themselves, and also in terms of how others see and engage with them.

This point about how one is viewed by others brings us to the topic of discrimination. For all of us, how we view ourselves, including our bodies, does not occur in a vacuum. Rather, it occurs in social contexts where particular bodies and ways of being are normalised, and others are treated at best as marginal, and at worst as deviant. Given the points about gender intensification outlined in the previous section, it is perhaps unsurprising that the period of adolescence brings with it for transgender young people not only increased self-scrutiny, but also increased scrutiny from others. Scrutinising one's self and body through a normative gendered lens constitutes an underlying mechanism for the phenomenology of dysphoria. Cisgenderism as an ideology instructs us as to what an appropriately gendered body should look and feel like in our particular cultural and historic context, thus meaning that for many transgender young people their bodies are experienced as diverging from their gender. Yet such self-scrutiny as it is informed by cisgenderism is greatly exacerbated by the scrutiny of others. The box below explores the topic of self-scrutiny with regard to the third case study.

Case Study 3: Necessary Actions

As a follow up to Tania's concerns about her female peers and questions about puberty, I initiated a conversation with Tania about what she wanted from the future. As is typical for many transgender young people, the present is often a central focus, and specifically on what is currently absent (i.e., hormones). I asked Tania what she thought puberty would bring. She understood that, for her, it would not bring menstruation. She could recognise that as for other people in her family of any gender, she had quite a shapely figure even at a young age, so she wasn't focused on that changing. Whilst she would be happy with breast growth, she didn't see that as a marker of her femininity, especially as she had an aunt who had her breasts removed due to cancer, and she could acknowledge that having no breasts did not make her aunt any less of a woman.

These conversations allowed Tania to explore how she had been scrutinising herself against a norm that didn't hold any inherent value to her. Certainly, questions from her female friends about puberty had triggered her concerns, but the questions she had been asked had been friendly enough, and hadn't been asked in a pejorative way (i.e., they didn't seem to have been aimed at belittling Tania for her lack of physical changes). Tania could actually acknowledge that she liked her body – it did what it needed to do, for now – and that she didn't need to compare herself to her female peers. This message of self-empowerment fitted well with Tania's own views on what it means to be a girl, and her mother's views on the need for girls and women to be resilient and resistant in the context of a male-dominated society that often encourages an over-focus on women and their bodies.

We know from the literature that transgender young people experience high rates of discrimination (see Grossman et al. 2011; Pullen Sansfaçon et al. 2018, for summaries). This can be from family members, from peers, from teachers, from healthcare professionals, and from strangers. All can perpetuate the cisgenderist narrative that there is something 'wrong' with transgender young people, including that their bodies are 'wrong'. This can be implicit – in the lack of inclusion or recognition of transgender young people – or it can be explicit, in acts of verbal and physical violence and exclusion. Transgender adolescents may be told or forced by their parents to conform to normative gendered expectations based on their assigned sex. They may be rejected outright by their parents. Their peers may ridicule them, intentionally misgender them, and refuse to associate with them. Strangers may target them for verbal harassment or physical abuse (as may family members and peers). For many transgender young people there are few places that are safe from discrimination, and places that may seem safe can become unsafe (such as we shall see, in Chap. 4, where parents may at first seem affirming, but later serve to undermine a transgender child). The box below explores how life became increasingly unsafe for Jordan.

> **Case Study 2: Distress Management**
> Despite the positive effects gained by commencing puberty blockers, Jordan reported experiencing an increasingly difficult time at school. He was now presenting as a boy at school and had asked his classmates and teachers to use the correct pronoun. However whilst his parents had supported him

accessing puberty blockers, they viewed using the correct pronouns (i.e., 'he') as a 'step too far', and again felt that should he 'change his mind' it would be much harder for everyone to change pronouns again. This lack of support from Ted and Julie meant that the school continued to waver in its support for Jordan. As a result, instances where Jordan was intentionally misgendered were not seen by the school as bullying, and Jordan had increasingly disengaged from school.

In many ways it felt to Jordan like the situation at school was beyond repair. Even if, somehow, his parents became supportive, he felt that the views of his peers were too entrenched for him to have a 'fresh start' within the school. As a result, we discussed the options available to Jordan. He was keen to finish school, and did not see leaving school as a viable option. We discussed other schools in the area but Jordan was concerned that he knew people at each school, and the problems with misgendering would continue. I mentioned that a number of other clients I work with are home schooled, though Jordan felt that being home all day with his mother and being taught by her would only further add to his distress. Jordan mentioned that he had recently visited his local library and had noticed that they had a study space there that could be booked for free. I suggested to Jordan that he could enrol in distance education and work in a self-directed way at the library. When we presented this idea to Julie and Ted, they were supportive, as it meant they did not have to confront the school and deal with trying to get the school to be supportive, but it also meant that Jordan would remain in education.

As I have emphasised throughout this chapter, this narrative of discrimination is not the only narrative to be told about transgender young people's lives. But it is most certainly a key narrative that represents the lives of many transgender young people, and as such it must be spoken about. This is particularly the case given what we know of the relationship between experiences of discrimination and poor mental health, suicidality, and self-harm (Holt et al. 2016). We know that many transgender young people living in the context of discrimination can see no way out. As such if, as clinicians, we do have the opportunity to work with transgender young people experiencing considerable distress (both due to dysphoria and/or discrimination), it is important that we have other narratives available to share with young people, as I will explore in the following section.

Puberty as a Time of Positive Growth

When I began to work with transgender adolescents over a decade ago, puberty blockers required court approval and most of the young people I worked with had little choice but to go through the puberty associated with their assigned sex. For most this brought considerable distress, and the extent of this distress often left us with little space in which to focus on adolescence as a time of positive growth. Certainly, sometimes we were able to explore topics such as dating and intimacy, but often even these were fraught by the overwhelmingness of dysphoria. In recent years, however, puberty blockers in Australia no longer require court approval (other than in cases where parents are not in agreement about treatment), making them much more accessible for a greater number of young people. As a result, I am seeing an increasing number of young people whose adolescence looks different to that described above. This is not to say that young people who are able to access puberty blockers and potentially hormones have an easy road: many still experience dysphoria, and many still experience discrimination. But it does mean that there can be greater clinical space in which to explore adolescence as a time of positive growth. An example of this is included in the box below.

Case Study 3: Distress Management

Despite our conversations about what Tania wanted for her future and that she did not need to accept stereotypes about what it means to be an adolescent girl, she remained concerned by what she perceived as her outsider status. In response to this, we had a conversation about what she thought was happening for other girls her age. Tania believed that they all had begun menstruating, and all wore bras and hence must have grown breasts. Tania also reported concern that whilst she wanted to be a mother one day, she feared that this would never happen due to being transgender.

Taking these concerns on board, we devised a plan. First, we returned to the difference between a secret and something that is private. We agreed that rather than Tania lying to her friends and saying she had started menstruating, she could simply say that it was private and she didn't feel comfortable talking about it. We discussed how her concerns about changing rooms could also be framed in the same way, and Tania acknowledged that some of the girls in her class also preferred to change in a cubicle.

In terms of breast growth, Tania's mother assured her that many of her peers would not have experienced breast growth, but instead would be wearing a bra with some padding. Tania was surprised to hear this, but could see how the norms about gender we had discussed previously can impact on everyone. She agreed that it wouldn't be deceptive or secretive for her to wear a bra with padding. We also spoke about the fact that she has begun puberty: she had become more mature over the many years that I had known her, and was more able to think through her feelings and discuss them. Tania felt happy that she could honestly say to her peers that she had 'begun puberty', without having to lie.

Finally, we discussed the opportunities available to Tania for parenthood. We discussed that scientific breakthroughs are on the horizon with regard to the creation of embryos from tissue (i.e., testicular or ovarian), rather than gametes. We also spoke about permanent foster care as options. And we spoke about potential partners who may well have their own gametes to use, in combination with donor gametes. Being able to talk through these options helped address the concerns that Tania had, and reduced her feelings of being an outsider.

There are four key areas indicated in the literature that speak to the topic of adolescence as a time of positive growth for transgender young people. These four areas are also reflected in my clinical work. The four areas are: (1) coming to a positive understanding of being transgender, (2) connecting in with other young people in online spaces, (3) the role of advocacy as a form of resilience, and (4) entering into the worlds of dating and intimacy. I now explore each of these in turn.

In terms of having a positive understanding of what it means to be transgender, it is important to first acknowledge that not all of the transgender young people I work with use the term 'transgender', or want to be known to others as transgender. This is nothing, in my experience, to do with shame, and everything to do with wanting to live a life just like their peers. This thinking can change with time, as some young people come to see a role for themselves as advocates, but for other young people this is not the case. Yet this is not to suggest that young people for whom the term 'transgender' is not their primary identity do not experience a positive understanding of what it means to be transgender. Indeed, across the diversity of young people I work with it is increasingly the case that being transgender is not seen as a cause of distress. This, in my experience, is a product of a subtle shift in public discourse, where young people are exposed to increasingly positive representations of transgender people in the media, and where to a certain extent public narratives are more inclusive or at least display awareness that transgender people exist.

For the young people surveyed in the Australian Trans Pathways report, many reported that being transgender allowed them to have an open mind, that it provided a sense of unity and pride, and that being transgender led them to a deep sense of self-awareness (Strauss et al. 2017). In other research transgender young people have similarly spoken about coming into a place of knowing about being transgender, and what this means for self-acceptance and positive growth. For example, the young people interviewed by Taylor (2015) reported a sense of empowerment through coming to understand dominant narratives about gender, and to be able to resist such narratives in their own self expressions, and to claim a space for themselves. For Taylor's participants, it wasn't that cisgenderism didn't occur, but rather that her participants felt empowered through their own growth and learning to resist the norms placed upon them, and to claim a positive sense of self as transgender. The topic of claiming a positive sense of self is explored in the box below.

Case Study 2: Ecologies of Support

In some ways counter to the GENDER case formulation, where ecologies of support refers to parties other than the transgender young person, for Jordan the most important form of support he could access was himself. This is, of course, entirely in line with a focus on self-growth within the mental health professions, and the need for all of us to be able to rely upon ourselves as a source of support. For Jordan, in the past the messages he had received from his parents had led to him question himself. The lack of support he had received at school meant that he felt that others perceived him as not worthy of friendship or support. Yet as we discussed, Jordan had shown considerable resilience in the face of such adversity. He had negotiated with his parents to start puberty blockers. He had negotiated to leave school and undertake distance education. These, I suggested, were the hallmarks of someone who is resilient, and who can effect change in their lives.

Focusing on the strengths that he displayed allowed Jordan to reconfigure how he saw himself. In visiting the library on a daily basis he had opportunities for new information to come in about himself. There he made friends, he socialised, and was viewed by others both as male, and as worthy of being shown care by others. By opening himself up to new information, and by starting with recognition of his own capacity for resilience and growth, Jordan was able to foster supportive networks that ushered in a new phase of growth in his life.

This point about self-expression relates to the second area identified in the literature, namely the vital role that online spaces can play for many transgender young people. Such spaces offer opportunities for young people to connect, to share information, and to develop safe and supportive networks. As Pollock and Eyre (2012) note in their research with transgender young men, seeing oneself in the stories of others can facilitate self-growth and understanding. Certainly for many of the young people I work with, as we shall see in the box below, hearing the stories of others, particularly in online spaces, has given them a language through which to describe their own feelings. Further, research suggests that online spaces can be a useful 'testing' ground for young people exploring their gender, and can lead to later in-person engagement that further contributes to positive growth (Pullen Sansfaçon et al. 2018). However, it is important to keep in mind that online spaces are not always safe for young people. The differing backgrounds and world views of transgender people means that there will be people who seek to enrich the lives of others, and people who may seek to negatively impact the lives of others. This is true for any community, and certainly in my experience can happen in the online spaces that transgender young people navigate. This means that clinicians have an important role to play in supporting transgender young people to develop critical literacy about online spaces, including setting their own boundaries, knowing when to disengage, and learning how to identify people who may wish them harm. None of this is to deny the important role that online spaces can play in facilitating connectedness for transgender young people, but it is to recognise that like any form of social interaction, they can also be spaces that require careful negotiation.

Case Study 3: Ecologies of Support

Despite her staunch position on not wanting to disclose that she is transgender to her peers, Tania increasingly desired to speak about her experiences with other young people. Francis shared that she was a part of a social media group for parents of transgender children, which she had found very meaningful and supportive. She informed Tania that the group

> has a private group for children, and that she was happy for Tania to join. Tania was excited by the idea that she might be able to speak with other transgender young people, and hear about their journeys, and particularly the ways in which they negotiate discussions about puberty. Tania and Francis agreed that at first Francis would sit with Tania to help her understand the social norms within the private group, and to ensure that she felt the space was safe.
>
> At a follow up appointment Tania reported that she had made two new friends – girls who lived locally to her. They had arranged that they would meet up in person with their parents, as they all desired to develop the friendships beyond online. For Tania, starting online had been a wonderful opportunity to come into a space where being transgender could be spoken about openly and honestly, with complete faith that any information would not be shared beyond the group. The degree of anonymity and separation had not only helped to build rapport with her new friends, but also trust. That all of their parents were in contact also helped to ensure that the new friendships were trustworthy.

In terms of the third area, self-advocacy can be important to many transgender young people. As noted above, some young people will not wish to speak publicly about being transgender, however research suggests that for many young people advocacy and public engagement further constitutes a possible form of positive growth. Research by Singh (2013), for example, suggests that advocacy constitutes a form of resilience enacted by many transgender young people in the face of discrimination. For some of Singh's participants, speaking out about their experiences, rallying for legislative or social change, and adopting a role as peer educators was an important form of resistance to contexts in which transgender young people are expected to be neither seen nor heard. As clinicians we have a role to play both as advocates ourselves, but also by facilitating or supporting the advocacy undertaken by the young people we work with. This can involve connecting young people in with advocacy groups, helping to identify key issues that require change, and working with young people to identify the barriers to advocacy and the importance of self-care in the face of potential opposition. The following box explores how Jordan, in collaboration with me, engaged in advocacy for another transgender young person.

> **Case Study 2: Reinforcement and Resistance**
>
> As Jordan developed new friendships, both online through his distance studies, and in person at the library, he was presented with opportunities to speak with trusted friends about being transgender. In particular, in speaking with one young person he learnt that their brother was also transgender. Jordan arranged to meet with this other young person, who was also having a difficult time with their family. For Jordan, being able to support another transgender young person was an important form of advocacy, and it allowed him to share all he had learnt through working with me and through his own growth.
>
> Jordan subsequently came to me asking for me to support his new friend, but it became apparent that the friend lived too far away, and that their parents were particularly resistant to their child seeing a clinician. Instead, Jordan and I identified a number of youth support groups that actively worked with transgender young people at risk of rejection or alienation by their parents. These groups also aimed to engage parents where possible. For Jordan this was another form of advocacy that reflected his growing confidence and capacity to effect positive change in the world around him.

The final area of positive growth connects to the literature on adolescence more broadly, specifically with regard to adolescence as a time of exploration of intimacy. As I noted above, for some transgender young people dysphoria may be a significant barrier to intimacy. Discrimination too can be a significant barrier to intimacy, particularly with regard to whether or not cisgender peers are capable of viewing transgender young people as intimate partners. Certainly the gender intensification hypothesis argues that early experiences of dating and intimacy can be formative in terms of the acceptance of gendered norms. For transgender young people, then, dating occurs in a context where potential intimate partners bring with them their own beliefs about gender which are likely impacted upon by social norms, and if these are particularly prescriptive and normative, then this can negatively impact upon transgender young people's experiences.

Yet both the research literature and clinical experience suggests that despite the challenges outlined above, many transgender young people successfully (to varying degrees) manage to negotiate the world of dating and intimacy. Some young people report that positive experiences of dating (where their gender is affirmed) can further reinforce their understanding of their gender and positively contribute to self-worth (Pullen Sansfaçon et al. 2018). From their interviews with young transgender men, Pollock and Eyre (2012) similarly report that experiences of intimacy affirmed their participants' gender. This was true for their heterosexual participants (e.g., "I think the first time I really kissed a girl was the first time I felt that I was male, truly. I just felt so male in that moment. It was a really powerful moment", p. 214) and their gay participants (e.g., "it took that validation [from gay men] for me to be like, 'Oh I actually do feel like I'm a guy'", p. 214). As is true for all adolescents, however, as clinicians we must be mindful that an over-focus on external validation in terms of dating can lead to problems. But this does not mean that we should not work with and support transgender young people who are exploring the worlds of dating and intimacy. Rather, it means supporting young people to engage in other-focused exploration *alongside* self-focused exploration, so that relationships with intimate partners becomes one part of personal growth, rather than the sole focus of personal growth.

Opening Up Spaces for Difficult Conversations

It might seem surprising, given the focus of the previous section on positive growth, to title this next section 'difficult conversations'. My suggestion in this section is that in order for clinicians to facilitate positive growth, sometimes we must have difficult conversations. These conversations may be difficult because they touch on dysphoria or discrimination. They may be difficult because they require deep thought. And they may be difficult because they speak to a future-orientation that may contradict a focus on the now. But in my clinical experience these can be important and powerful conversations, from which many transgender young people experience considerable growth.

A key difficult conversation I frequently have with the young people I work with relates to what kind of person they will be when they grow up. Often, when I ask an adolescent boy what kind of man he will be, this is heard as questioning his gender. This is understandable, given that for many of the young people I work with they are indeed questioned about their gender. In my framing of the question, however, I emphasise that there are many different ways to be a particular gender. One can, for example, be a kind man who respects women and animals, or a man who thinks everyone should bow to his wishes. In asking about what type of person they might be with regard to their gender, then, my focus is thus not on their career plans or life-long ambitions. Rather, it is to ask the young people I work with to think about gender norms and stereotypes, and to appreciate that who they will grow up to be in regards to gender can be intentionally shaped, provided they are mindful about their understanding of gender.

If we think back to the literature on adolescence, we can appreciate that the gender intensification hypothesis may explain to a certain extent how and why differences between girls and boys are exhibited. For transgender young people, and depending on their social circles and other influences such as family, this can mean they either experience broad exposure to a variety of ways that people inhabit and enact their gender, or a limited variety. Given that the gender intensification hypothesis emphasises how social interactions serve to indoctrinate or normalise particular ways of doing gender (that, given, cisgenderism, are most commonly linked to assumptions about assigned sex), then for transgender young people their exposure to norms around gender will often be limited to other people's assumptions about their gender. Coming into an understanding of one's gender, then, does not automatically mean that all transgender young people will know what others expect of their gender, and indeed even if they do, it is likely that their understanding will be normative. The types of questions that I ask young people, then, are aimed at opening up the space for conversations about what they know about gender as a category, not about questioning their gender. The questions are aimed at challenging the stereotypes that some young people may feel they need to conform to, and to raise awareness about the many ways they can live their gender.

Having difficult conversations about what it means to live one's gender can result in many outcomes. It can lead to some young people reaffirming a very normative understanding of their gender. It can mean that girls who enjoy wearing dresses and who want to be mothers when they grow up continue to do so. Difficult conversations can also lead to change. For some young men it has helped prepare them for what others will expect of them – that female partners, for example, may want them to adopt a particular role in a relationship – and to know how to resist the expectations of others. For other young men it has helped draw attention to the relative privilege that (most) men hold in male-dominated societies, and to be mindful of the invitations they will receive to enact this privilege in harmful ways. For some young women it has involved having conversations about misogyny, and what this can look like for transgender women specifically. Across all of these conversations my aim is never to promote one particular way of being any given gender. Rather, it is about encouraging a critical lens on gender norms, so that young people feel able to express themselves in whatever way feels right for them, always mindful of social norms and expectations.

Related to these conversations about gender are conversations about sexuality. For many of the young people I work with, the message they receive from those around them with regard to intimacy and attractions is heteronormative. This can mean that when they come to enter the world of dating and intimacy, they may feel that the only way to express their gender is to be attracted to someone of a different gender to them. Yet we know from the literature that many transgender people experience a diverse range of sexualities, and that whilst historically heterosexuality was the expected and indeed mandated pathway for transgender people seeking medical transition, respecting and affirming transgender people's sexualities beyond heterosexuality is vital. For some young people I have worked with, who have voiced that they are heterosexual, over time and through our conversations about gender, they have come to recognise that their attractions are more diverse, as we shall see in the box below. This is not to suggest that my role has been to advocate for a broadening of attractions. Rather, my role is to create a safe space in which young people can explore a range of emotions and attractions, rather than feeling limited by normative assumptions about who they should be attracted to (if anyone).

Case Study 3: Reinforcement and Resistance

Of all the challenges faced by Tania, one of the greatest was the topic of intimacy. In our conversations about motherhood, Tania had skirted around the possibility that she might be in a relationship when she sought to become a mother. As I learnt, this skirting – and Tania's concerns about motherhood in general – were related to her as yet unexpressed attraction to other girls. It wasn't that she thought her parents wouldn't accept this. Rather, she thought that everyone expected a transgender girl to be attracted to boys, and that being attracted to girls would lead other people to question whether or not she was transgender. When this topic presented itself, I was able to engage in a frank and honest discussion with Tania about the legitimacy of her feelings, validating her growing sense of attraction to other girls. We spoke about how she thought intimacy would look for her, her degree of comfort with her body, and a particular trusted and much cared for friend whom she had met through the private online group.

For Tania, as we moved through these conversations, she become increasingly vocal about the fact that one day she might want to speak to others about being transgender. She felt that some of the worries and stressors she had experienced were a result of not knowing. She was thankful for her parents, but also came to see that both parents and children don't know what they don't know. Her parents hadn't known to speak with her about the legitimacy of whatever attractions she felt. For Tania, she felt that one day in the future, there might be an important advocacy role for her to play in speaking with other girls about 'being whoever they want to be'.

Related to conversations about sexuality and intimacy are conversations about bodies. As I explored earlier in this chapter, for many transgender young people dysphoria can limit how much they are willing to talk or think about their bodies. And certainly these limitations must be respected. But we also know from the literature that re-gendering normative understandings of bodies can play an important role in reducing dysphoria. This can include transgender boys and young men speaking about their genitalia using terms such as 'dick', or 'penis' or 'front hole' (Edelman and Zimman 2014; Riggs and Bartholomaeus 2018). This re-gendering of genitalia can open up possibilities for conversations about intimacy that were previously closed due to dysphoria. A useful focus can also include conversations about function that resists normative assumptions. So, for example, public narratives about gender transition that utilise the language of 'sex change' fundamentally misunderstand what 'changes' about bodies. For many transgender men, phalloplasty may be unaffordable, or unavailable. Yet for many transgender men (including adolescents) hormone therapies are much more available. Testosterone can produce significant changes to genitalia that change their function for transgender men, something that many young people are not aware of when they begin thinking about intimacy. Similarly, for young women who are exploring intimacy, practices such as 'muffing' offer opportunities for intimacy that may not be generally discussed. Clinicians have an important role to play in opening up difficult conversations about bodies and intimacy, and sharing resources on the topic that are written by and for transgender people (e.g., Bellwether 2010; Pez 2013).

Concluding Thoughts

A growing narrative within transgender communities is a shift from the language of dysphoria to one of euphoria. Gender euphoria refers to the elation and positive growth that results from coming into a place of "positive gender fulfillment" (Benestad 2010, p. 227). Such a shift is important, as it acknowledges that public narratives of transgender people's lives that in the past and still in the present have emphasised sadness and distress are not the only narratives possible. With regard to young people specifically, Roen (2018) questions how narratives of distress and trauma, as they predominate in the literature, direct some transgender young people towards particular negative pathways, and indeed that distress is seen as a required part of being transgender. My argument in this chapter is that in some ways we need an understanding of both gender dysphoria and euphoria, and this is because of cisgenderism. Cisgenderism means that some young people *will* feel dysphoric about their bodies, but at the same time some young people will resist cisgenderism, or re-gender and re-narrate their bodies and lives in ways that are affirming.

As clinicians we have an important role to play in both listening to and acknowledging dysphoria, and also engaging in conversations that promote positive growth that may engender a sense of gender euphoria. These conversations, as I elaborated above, are sometimes necessarily difficult, and it is important that we balance out the wellbeing of the young person with the potential utility of having these conversations. Some young people may not be in a place where they can have difficult conversations. But the astute clinician can identify moments where a difficult question can be asked safely, and left for the young person to think about. Sometimes a question I ask in one session may not be engaged with by a young person until many sessions later, once they've had time to process the question and feel safe to engage with it. Our ability as clinicians to ask difficult questions is directly shaped by cisgenderism, and the degree to which it is directing the lives of the young people we work with. As such, a central component to our work must always be to challenge cisgenderism in our daily lives, so as to work alongside transgender young people to create worlds where cisgenderism does not so completely rule all of our lives, and so that our conversations about adolescence, gender, change, and growth can become more possible. This is a topic to which I will return in the final chapter of this book.

References

American Psychiatric Association. (2013). *Diagnostic and statistical manual of mental disorders (DSM-5)*. Washington, DC: American Psychiatric Association.
Bellwether, M. (2010). *Fucking trans women*. Retrieved June 8, 2018, from http://fuckingtranswomen.org
Benestad, E. E. P. (2010). From gender dysphoria to gender euphoria: An assisted journey. *Sexologies, 19*(4), 225–231.
De Vries, A. L., McGuire, J. K., Steensma, T. D., Wagenaar, E. C., Doreleijers, T. A., & Cohen-Kettenis, P. T. (2014). Young adult psychological outcome after puberty suppression and gender reassignment. *Pediatrics, 134*(4), 696–704.
Edelman, E. A., & Zimman, L. (2014). Boycunts and bonus holes: Trans men's bodies, neoliberalism, and the sexual productivity of genitals. *Journal of Homosexuality, 61*(5), 673–690.
Faust, M. S. (1983). Alternative constructions of adolescent growth. In J. Brooks-Gunn & A. C. Petersen (Eds.), *Girls at puberty: Biological and psychosocial perspectives* (pp. 105–125). Boston: Springer.

Grossman, A. H., D'Augelli, A. R., & Frank, J. A. (2011). Aspects of psychological resilience among transgender youth. *Journal of LGBT Youth, 8*(2), 103–115.

Hill, J. P., & Lynch, M. E. (1983). The intensification of gender-related role expectations during early adolescence. In J. Brooks-Gunn & A. C. Petersen (Eds.), *Girls at puberty: Biological and psychosocial perspectives* (pp. 201–228). Boston: Springer.

Holt, V., Skagerberg, E., & Dunsford, M. (2016). Young people with features of gender dysphoria: Demographics and associated difficulties. *Clinical Child Psychology and Psychiatry, 21*(1), 108–118.

Lesko, N. (2012). *Act your age! A cultural construction of adolescence* (2nd ed.). New York: Routledge.

McGuire, J. K., Doty, J. L., Catalpa, J. M., & Ola, C. (2016). Body image in transgender young people: Findings from a qualitative, community based study. *Body Image, 18*, 96–107.

Pez, J. (2013). *Dude magazine*. Retrieved June 8, 2018, from https://dudemagazine.wordpress.com/download-issues/

Pollock, L., & Eyre, S. L. (2012). Growth into manhood: Identity development among female-to-male transgender youth. *Culture, Health & Sexuality, 14*(2), 209–222.

Pullen Sansfaçon, A., Hébert, W., Lee, E. O. J., Faddoul, M., Tourki, D., & Bellot, C. (2018). Digging beneath the surface: Results from stage one of a qualitative analysis of factors influencing the well-being of trans youth in Quebec. *International Journal of Transgenderism, 19*(2), 184–202.

Riggs, D. W., & Bartholomaeus, C. (2018). Transgender young people's narratives of intimacy and sexual health: Implications for sexuality education. *Sex Education, 18*(4), 376–390.

Roen, K. (2018). Rethinking queer failure: Trans youth embodiments of distress. *Sexualities*. https://doi.org/10.1177/1363460717740257.

Singh, A. A. (2013). Transgender youth of color and resilience: Negotiating oppression and finding support. *Sex Roles, 68*(11–12), 690–702.

Strauss, P., Cook, A., Winter, S., Watson, V., Wright Toussaint, D., & Lin, A. (2017). *Trans pathways: The mental health experiences and care pathways of trans young people*. Telethon Kids Institute, Perth.

Taylor, G. L. (2015). *Being trans: An interpretative phenomenological study of young adults*. Unpublished Honours Thesis, Edith Cowan University.

4

Parent Journeys Through Cisgenderism

Reading the literature on parents of transgender children can be challenging. It is a literature dominated by a narrative wherein parents are depicted as having to make a journey as a result of having a transgender child, a journey marked by loss, distress, challenges and fears. In this chapter my aim is to unpack why it is that these narratives are so prevalent. Ultimately, my argument is that cisgenderism as the backdrop to parenting creates a context wherein transgender children are widely viewed as challenges or losses to parents. More specifically, narratives of loss, as I have suggested elsewhere (Bartholomaeus and Riggs 2017; Riggs and Bartholomaeus 2018a, b), are a product of parents feeling that they have lost ready access to the 'easy life' they presumed they had as a result of cisgenderism (a life in which most parents assume that their child will be cisgender). In response to such negative framings, in this chapter I offer an alternate framing, one that acknowledges the many emotions that parents may experience, but which focuses on how cisgenderism produces such emotions, rather than transgender children themselves. Doing so is important as it takes the focus away from the child (and thus reduces the likelihood that children will be blamed or responded to in ways that are not affirming), and instead places the focus squarely on the norms that parents must negotiate with in order to come to a place where they can be affirming.

Developmentally, the broader literature suggests that parents influence their children with regard to gender expression in four ways. Owen Blakemore, Berenbaum and Liben (2009) summarise these as (1) parents channelling or shaping their children's gendered interests, (2) differential treatment of children according to their gender, (3) direct instruction from parents about what boys or girls are supposed to do, and (4) parents modelling gendered behaviours and roles. In this chapter I use this framework from the developmental literature on gender through which to read the literature on parents of transgender children. As has been the case with other chapters in this book, this allows me to, in places, challenge the cisgenderism of the developmental literature, but also to account for the concerns above with regard to how transgender children are positioned. Importantly, however, in this chapter I also explore research where parents resist cisgenderism, instead finding ways to celebrate their transgender child following disclosure, or indeed prior to disclosure via critical understandings of normative gender ideologies.

Parents and Children's Gender Expression

In the subsections that follow I summarise the four ways in which parents may influence their children with regard to gender. Drawing on Chap. 2, however, I would note that in many ways what is being accounted for both in the literature on parents of transgender children, and the literature on parents and gender development more broadly, is how parents may influence how children *express* their gender. Whilst, as discussed in Chap. 2, how parents engage with or narrate the categories that children bring with them as they acquire spoken language will shape children's gendered understandings, children's sense of themselves as inhabiting a particular category will already be in place. This is not to deny that parents can have an influence on how children see themselves. Rather, it is to acknowledge that very young children make agentic decisions about themselves, even if those decisions may then be shaped by the responses they receive from their parents. The focus in this first section of the chapter, then, is on how parents may shape transgender children's gender expression, and more specifically, how they may refuse to acknowledge it due to cisgenderism. In the box below I outline the first part of a case where the parents of a transgender child were struggling to acknowledge their child's gender.

> **Case Study 4: Gender Journey and Understanding**
>
> Trudy and her husband Mark scheduled an appointment with me to speak about their child's gender. Early in the appointment they spoke about their 11 year old male assigned child, Andrew, an only child whom they described as being very feminine, and who they thought was probably gay. I asked them why they had come to see me, given I specialise in working with transgender children, not gay children *per se* (acknowledging, of course, that transgender children can be gay). Mark admitted that they had come to see me because they were worried that their child wasn't gay but rather was transgender, and they 'wanted to do something about that'. As Mark said, he could, in time, come to handle his child being gay, but he couldn't accept his child being transgender.
>
> Trudy was quiet throughout the session, and after the session ended she emailed me to let me know that she was very worried for her child. Her child had become increasingly withdrawn, and often seemed scared of Mark. Trudy noted that she felt she had little capacity to stand up to Mark's views on transgender children, and didn't know where to turn. She had her own problems in her relationship with Mark, and felt they were now spilling out onto Andrew.

Also important to note is that my focus in this chapter (and throughout this book) is on cisgender parents of transgender children. Transgender parents may, of course, raise transgender children, and transgender parents also raise children in the context of cisgenderism. However, my aim in this chapter is to focus on parents who are most likely to present to clinicians in terms of needing assistance in coming to understand and celebrate a transgender child. Certainly, transgender parents may benefit from engaging with clinicians, but it is less likely that this will be a product of struggling to affirm a transgender child.

Parents Channelling or Shaping Their Children's Gendered Interests

Channelling or shaping refers primarily to parents directing children towards interests or activities that are normatively gendered. This means, for example, giving trucks to children assigned male, or dolls to children assigned female. As I discussed in Chap. 2, this type of channelling as discussed in the developmental literature typically presumes that directing a child's play towards interests normatively associated with their assigned sex will directly shape their gender. However, we know that for many children this assumption is not the case, and more broadly that it limits *all* children's understandings of their own and other people's genders. In the developmental literature in general, studies have found that parents are increasingly accepting of female assigned children who engage in a diverse range of gendered play, yet a majority of parents still are adverse to accepting such diverse play amongst children assigned male (e.g., Kane 2006). As we shall now see, this has specific implications for transgender children.

In her interviews with 24 parents of 'gender variant' children, Rahilly (2015) found that a majority engaged in what she terms 'gender hedging'. Gender hedging, Rahilly suggests, was one way in which parents sought to minimise or deny their child's gender diversity, specifically with regards to clothing, toys, and activities. For some of Rahilly's participants, they made small concessions aimed at curtailing the 'spread' of gender diversity (e.g., by buying pink socks for a child assigned male, but refusing to buy a doll for the same child). Other participants reported allowing clothing stereotypically associated with the child's gender (rather than assigned sex) at home, but not allowing them to wear such clothing outside of the home. Elsewhere I have discussed how parents may use this distinction between 'at home' and 'outside' clothes as a means to gaslighting transgender children (Riggs and Bartholomaeus 2018a, b). Gaslighting is a form of emotional control whereby a person blames their own negative actions upon the person who is subject to the actions. So, for example, Rahilly suggests that for some of her participants, rather than acknowledging that they were not willing to affirm a transgender child in terms of clothing, they would blame the child for their 'sloppy' presentation, thus justifying their refusal to support the wearing of specific items of clothing.

In a different way, the research of Ryan (2016) also examines how parents may channel or shape transgender children's gender expression through clothing or toys. From her interviews with 36 mothers of gender diverse young people, Ryan reports that a majority of her participants were 'gender expansive', in that they were parents who previously had no understanding of gender diversity, but whose understandings of gender had 'expanded' as a result of raising a gender diverse child. Yet such expansion was often still limited by cisgenderist understandings of gender expression. Ryan provides two specific examples: one of a mother who persisted with the framing that there are 'girl things' and 'boy things', but insisted that any person can like either, the other a mother who reframed all clothing and toys as gender neutral. Ryan suggests that the first framing is problematic, in that whilst it accepts that any child can like any 'thing', there is still a 'correct' thing to like, and that is determined by one's gender (or more specifically, by one's assigned sex which is presumed to determine gender). The box below introduces a second case study that focuses on a parent who may be seen as 'gender expansive'. I would suggest further that the second framing may also be problematic. Reframing all clothing and toys as gender neutral may be less than affirming for binary transgender children who see normatively gendered clothing or toys as a way to reflect their gender to the world around them.

Case Study 5: Gender Journey and Understanding

Lucy, aged 7, came to see me with her mother Annika, who was a single parent to Lucy and her brother Jake. Annika was effusive from the beginning of the first session about Lucy being transgender, noting with joy that she had grown so much as a parent following Lucy's disclosure a year earlier. Annika grew up in a relatively conservative household, but as an adult she has had many opportunities to expand her horizons in terms of how she thinks about the world, and felt that affirming Lucy was a logical next step in this growth.

Half way through the session Lucy seized on a pause in the conversation to share her own thoughts. She was thankful that her mother had been so affirming, which had included supporting her to change her name legally, to change schools so that she could have a 'fresh start', and advocating for Lucy in terms of family members being affirming and using her name and the correct pronouns. I asked Jake how he felt in terms of supporting his sister, and he stated that he loved having a sister.

In contrast to the potential problem with treating all clothing and toys as gender neutral, Wren's (2002) interviews with 11 parents of transgender children suggests that for some of her participants early interests in toys or activities not normatively associated with a child's assigned sex were retrospectively viewed as 'proof' that a child was transgender. Certainly this type of logic reflects the diagnostic tools contained in the DSM5 (American Psychiatric Association 2013), where one of the criterion for a diagnosis of gender dysphoria in children is "a strong preference for toys, games, or activities stereotypically used or engaged in by the other gender" (p. 452). Yet this logic is problematic both for parents and in the context of the DSM5, in that it treats 'preferences' as indicative of gender. Whilst I suggested above that for some transgender children normatively gendered toys or clothing may be an important signifier of their gender, this will not be the case for all children. Treating toys and clothing as a key signifier, then, is problematic as it limits our capacity to affirm children's gender expressions, and indeed to acknowledge that a child may be transgender. The box below explores in more detail how a focus on channelling and shaping became a key source of stress for Trudy and her child.

Case Study 4: Expressed Concerns

At our next appointment Trudy came alone, and informed me that following her email correspondence Mark had done a 'sweep' of the house and removed any toys or items that he deemed to be 'too girlie'. This included some cars that had the colour pink on them, a dress up that was seen to be 'ambiguous', and a number of books with female protagonists. This clean out, which occurred when no one else was home, resulted in their child running away from home for a four hour period, which left Trudy in considerable distress, but which left Mark even more resolute that they needed to 'fix this problem right now'.

When Trudy managed to locate her child at a friend's house nearby, Trudy decided that she would take some time out from Mark and stay with her child at her sister's house. In the week after she left Mark sent over 100 threatening messages, leading to Trudy taking their child out of school for fear that Mark might retaliate and take their child. Trudy reported that her child had been somewhat happy once away from Mark, but was also fearful about what would happen if Mark managed to regain access.

Differential Treatment of Children According to Their Gender

In the literature on gender development differential treatment refers to treating children assigned male and children assigned female differently, according to assumptions about the inherent interests and emotions of each group of children. So, for example, researchers have examined how mothers may encourage their female assigned children to emote or may be more concerned about their emotional wellbeing, whereas mothers of male assigned children may encourage them to minimise their emotions and may pay less attention to their emotional wellbeing (Rosen, Adamson and Bakeman 1992). This type of normative gendered differential treatment is problematic for all children, but specifically problematic for transgender children given the ways in which it likely closes down the ways in which children may express their gender (albeit in ways regulated by normative assumptions, though as I noted above, for some children this may be an important way of claiming their gender).

In many ways these types of assumptions about differential treatment constitute a form of biological essentialism, whereby parents assume that a child's assigned sex should determine how they should be treated by their parents (e.g., that female assigned children will be more 'delicate', and male assigned child will be more 'robust'). Certainly in the literature on parents of transgender children, an investment in biological essentialism appears to be a key indicator of when parents might narrate a transgender child as a 'loss'. In her interviews with 37 people who had a transgender family member (a majority of whom were parents of transgender children), Norwood (2013) reported that a majority drew upon biological essentialist arguments to frame a transgender family member as a loss, given the assumption that someone who transitions gender 'replaces' the person who came before. Whilst arguments about biological essentialism did not prevent these participants from, in varying ways, coming to affirm their transgender family member, a reliance upon biological essentialism produced a feeling of loss. In other words, when someone is presumed to be one gender, but then discloses that they are a different gender, the logic of 'replacement' produces a narrative of loss.

This is a particularly nuanced version of cisgenderism, in that not only is it about the presumption that assigned sex determines gender, but more specifically that knowing someone's gender is widely considered central to knowing *who they are* (i.e., it is viewed as a higher order identity category that is commonly oriented to when we cognitively sort people into groups when we meet them, itself a product of cisgenderism).

> **Case Study 5: Expressed Concerns**
> At the end of the first session Lucy asked if she might see me on her own, and Annika was very supportive of this. At our one-on-one session Lucy reported that she was a little worried about how exuberant her mother was. Lucy felt that whilst she was very thankful that her mother was so affirming, she nonetheless felt that this left little space in which she could explore or express her gender. Lucy noted that Annika was very stereotypically feminine in her gender presentation, and when Lucy had disclosed that she was transgender Annika had rushed out and bought her a range of 'princess dresses'. Lucy felt like she was required to be a 'little Annika', which didn't speak to how Lucy experienced her gender.
> Lucy also felt that Annika had made a marked shift in how she engaged with her. Previously, Lucy had enjoyed a range of activities including sports, however upon disclosing to Annika that she was transgender Lucy had been directed towards other activities that were more stereotypically feminine. Lucy felt that this had distanced her from her closest friends (many of whom were boys), and made her feel isolated.

In other research, such narratives of loss are managed through recourse to exactly the kinds of assumptions about differential treatment that produce the narratives in the first place. In her interviews with 14 parents of transgender children, for example, Aramburu Alegría (2018) found that for many of her participants one way they came to terms with a child being transgender was to very rapidly shift their gendered thinking. In other words, these participants sought to quickly replace one logic for differential treatment with another, limited strictly to a gender binary, as one participant stated: "if he is going to be a boy, then he needs to be a masculine boy, not girly" (p. 142). As Meadow (2018) notes: "Parents… can move an individual child from one category to another, and the entire apparatus [of gender], all the social processes previously employed to shore up an individual child as male, then shift to consolidate the very same person as female" (p. 9). Dealing with feelings of loss by insisting upon a simple binary change in thinking about gender appears to allow such parents to continue on with a logic of differential treatment that potentially does very little to actually listen to how transgender children narrate their gender.

Direct Instruction from Parents About What Boys or Girls Are Supposed to Do

Reference to direct instruction in the literature in terms of gender development in some ways overlaps with differential treatment, but also constitutes a distinct way in which parents may regulate their children's gender expression. In terms of overlaps, direct instruction might involve telling male assigned children that 'boys don't cry', which is also a form of differential treatment (i.e., attending to the emotions of female assigned children but minimising the emotions of male assigned children). Both direct instruction and differential treatment, then, are about biological essentialism. Yet direct instruction can take different forms to differential treatment, in that it is typically explicit rather than implicit. Explicit direct instruction can be as 'simple' as saying 'you are a good boy' (thus giving an explicit message about what gender a child is presumed to be), or it can be more 'complex', such as saying 'boys can't do ballet' (thus making a generalisation about an entire category of people to which a child is presumed to belong). Along with channelling and shaping, direct instruction is often a key way in which transgender children's gender expression is limited by parents.

Returning to the work of Wren (2002), for some of her participants direct instruction took the form of parents insisting that a child was not transgender, rather that they were too immature to know their gender and instead needed further direct instruction about how to be the gender normatively associated with their assigned sex. This is a concern explored further in the box below. Certainly this type of parenting does not come out of nowhere. Rather, it is exactly the type of clinical response that many parents would have received by clinicians wedded to a 'curative' (i.e., non-affirming) approach to transgender children. The first child I ever worked with came to me, along with her parents, in great distress, because a clinician had told the family to burn the child's dresses and send her to an all boys school. Furthermore, and echoing the material covered above with regard to channelling and shaping, parents may gaslight a child in terms of direct instruction. They may, for example, tell their child that going against their direct instruction and wearing clothing that reflects their gender is a 'safety risk', and that in order to 'be safe' they need to follow their parents' rules about what clothes they can and cannot wear.

> **Case Study 4: Necessary Actions**
>
> At our next appointment Trudy came along with her child, who she was now calling 'Drew', at their request. At the appointment Trudy was searching for ways to understand her child, and was especially focused on how an 11 year old can know themselves enough to know their gender. I asked Trudy what she was like at age 11. Did she know then that she was a girl? Trudy struggled to answer this question, her only response being that she knew what genitalia she had, so she guessed that meant she knew what her gender was. Though our conversations Trudy had come to appreciate that genitalia don't determine gender, but she was still stuck on the idea that Drew could know their gender.
>
> I reflected to Trudy that in many ways her concerns about maturity were on a spectrum with Mark's seemingly more extreme views. Questioning Drew's capacity to know their gender was not the same as disposing of toys or being aggressive, but it was still part of a broader narrative where children's views are seen as unreliable. I encouraged Drew and Trudy to speak about what gender means to be them: what it means to experience themselves as being a particular gender, and what it means when that experience is not heard. Trudy was able to reflect upon how, for most of their relationship, Mark had been highly regulatory of her gender expression, not allowing her to cut her hair, and questioning her when she wore clothes that he read as even slightly masculine. Trudy left the appointment with a commitment to working through her own assumptions about gender in relation to Drew.

Importantly, however, parents who are affirming of a transgender child may simply seek to substitute one form of direct instruction for another (Meadow 2011). Returning to Ryan's (2016) work on 'gender expansive' mothers, she argues that some of her participants were happy to reframe a male assigned child as 'a girl with a penis', yet the emphasis in such a statement very much was 'girl', bringing with it a range of direct instructions about what girls can and cannot do. For these mothers, then, whilst the 'expanding' of their understanding of gender afforded them opportunities to affirm diversity in terms of gender-as-being, it did not necessarily allow for an expansion of their understandings of gender expression. Certainly, as I noted above, for some transgender children there may be a desire for direct instruction normatively associated with their gender, and this may be experienced as affirming. But this will not be the case for all transgender children, and more broadly it does take into account that such normative direct instruction may be limiting for all transgender children.

Parents Modelling Gendered Behaviours and Roles

Finally in terms of how parents may regulate a child's gender expression, modelling refers to the ways in which parents, as gendered beings, demonstrate to children how to be a particular gender. So, for example, in a cisgender heterosexual-headed household where a mother cares for children and engages in part-time paid work around her parenting responsibilities, and the father engages in full-time paid work and very little child care or house work, this models to children what men or women are expected to do. The topic of modelling is explored in more detail in the box below. For parents of transgender children, I would argue, the logic that underpins modelling (i.e., that children normatively reflect back to parents their own gendered roles) serves yet again to produce loss. In other words, when a child does *not* reflect back to a parent a normative sense of their gender, then this can leave parents questioning what they have done (i.e., have they failed to correctly model their gender for their child). Again, this type of logic is not surprising, given that pathologising approaches to transgender children have typically blamed parents (and specifically 'overly attached mothers' and 'absent fathers'). Importantly, then, the loss that parents may experience is not a product of their child, but rather a product of their own investment in social norms that instruct parents as to how their modelling should be reflected by their child in terms of gender (and indeed sexuality with regard to heteronormativity).

> **Case Study 5: Necessary Actions**
>
> At our next appointment Annika and Lucy came together. At our one-on-one appointment Lucy and I had developed a number of strategies for how we might respectfully challenge Annika in her thinking about gender expression. Key to this was a distinction between gender-as-being and gender expression. Lucy was more than articulate in the session with Annika in terms of saying 'look, Mum, I know I am a girl, but there are lots of ways to be a girl'. Annika at first was shocked by the idea that she might have 'gotten something wrong'. She felt she had tried so hard to be affirming, and had done everything she could think of to support Lucy.
>
> Lucy and I reflected to Annika that her views on what constitutes being affirming are likely shaped by her own views on being a woman. Annika could admit that, as a single mother, she felt very responsible for 'how her children turned out', and that she was mindful that other people might blame her for the fact that Lucy is transgender. She wanted to help Lucy be the best girl she could be, but was able to see that this type of thinking had limited her understanding of what it meant for Lucy, instead focusing on her own motivations as a mother. We ended the session with a commitment from Annika to work on listening to Lucy in terms of how she wishes to express her gender.

Across the literature on parents of transgender children there are multiple examples of how parents manage how other people may hold them to account for having a transgender child (and thus what this says about them as parents and about their gender). Gregor et al. (2015), for example, in their interviews with eight parents of transgender children, report that many framed being transgender as a product of having a 'faulty' gene, which both positioned them as responsible (i.e., the child was a product of their genetics), yet provided a plausible explanation (i.e., one's genetics are beyond one's control). The 60 parents surveyed in an earlier study I conducted also largely reported viewing gender as biologically-determined, and hence having a transgender child was not a product of parenting but rather destiny (Riggs and Due 2015). Some of the 49 parents interviewed by Meadow (2011) made recourse to lay understandings of epigenetics in order to explain environmental factors as playing a role in a child being transgender. Finally, some of Norwood's (2013) participants argued that gender was psychological rather than biological but that whilst one's psychology is a product of many factors, it is nonetheless rooted in an internal truth that is not subject to outside influence.

As Rahilly (2015) has argued, all of the types of accounts outlined above do very little to move beyond biological essentialism, hence perpetuating the very logic that produces a sense of loss for some parents in the first place. Moreover, and as was the case for the other forms of parental influence upon gender expression outlined above, such accounts simply replace a narrative of loss with a narrative of certainty. In other words, when a child discloses that they are transgender, a parent, by drawing on the biological essentialist narratives outlined above, can account for this through recourse to biology, and then simply 'switch' role models (in heterosexual-headed families where a transgender child has a binary gender). Rather than challenging the cisgenderism that produces narratives of loss, then, this account of modelling perpetuates it. We might consider, for example, what might happen if a transgender child with a binary gender later discloses that they have a non-binary gender. I certainly see this in my practice, where over time and through being affirmed a child feels comfortable to explore gender beyond binary categories. Being wedded to a binary understanding of gender as a way to respond to feelings of loss doesn't equip parents with the capacity to see gender in other ways (and indeed may serve to gate keep children's own gendered understandings and explorations). This was certainly the case in one of the cases I outline in this chapter, as we shall see in the box below.

> **Case Study 4: Distress Management**
> I was somewhat surprised to receive an email from Mark asking for an appointment, and was somewhat apprehensive about seeing Mark alone. From all reports Trudy and Drew were living in fear of Mark, however it seemed important to try and listen to how Mark was processing things. During the appointment Mark appeared relatively calm, however nonetheless was very wedded to his view that genitalia determines gender, and that he could never accept Drew being anything other than a boy. I pointed out to Mark that he had used the name 'Drew', and he reflected on the fact that it was a 'neutral' name, so it didn't bother him too much.
> Building on this reflection, I suggested to Mark that perhaps part of the problem he was facing was that he was so wedded to gender as a binary that he wasn't able to hear what Drew was saying in terms of their gender. My point was not to minimise Drew's gender journey, but rather to mitigate Mark's poorly informed views about transgender children and a diver-

> sity of gender expressions. Mark often referenced highly normative and pathologising images of transgender people he had seen in the media, and he couldn't conceptualise a life for his child beyond that. I suggested that what we needed was to actually listen to Drew, rather than make assumptions about Drew's gender.

Parents Challenging Cisgenderism

As I noted in the introduction to this chapter, much of the literature on parents of transgender children focuses on narratives of loss, distress, challenges, and fear. We can see an example of this in the box below. Yet there is a growing body of literature that focuses on parents who resist or simply do not experience these narratives, and instead who affirm a transgender child from the onset. As I will summarise in this section, some of this literature focuses less on critical accounts of gender development, and more on the important role that parents can play in affirming their children in terms of their wellbeing. Other literature, however, very much critically investigates how some parents actively challenge cisgenderism and normative gender ideologies. I now consider each of these literatures in turn.

> **Case Study 5: Distress Management**
> At our next appointment Annika came on her own, as she wanted to share some concerns. She had reflected on how imposing her views on gender expression on Lucy was less than helpful for Lucy, but she was also worried that if Lucy didn't present as normatively feminine then people would not accept her. Annika noted that whilst she had for a moment felt that she had 'lost' a child she thought was male when Lucy first disclosed that she was transgender, she quickly came to see that 'all would be fine' as Annika 'knows what it means to be female' and could share this with Lucy. In terms of Lucy's gender expression, then, Annika was concerned given her perception that normative gender expression is a gateway to inclusion, and Annika felt that the best she could do to affirm Lucy was to facilitate her inclusion in the social world through a normative expression of femininity.
> I reflected to Annika that girls express themselves in a diversity of ways, and that in most cases this does not prevent them having meaningful and supportive relationships with other people. We also spoke about the intersections of inclusion and self worth, and that being included by presenting yourself in a way that you think other people will like isn't necessarily a

route to a strong sense of self worth. Annika could see that for so much of her life her self worth had hinged on her femininity, and that this had been limiting for her. She didn't want this for Lucy.

In terms of the literature that focuses on parents affirming a transgender child, research by Durwood, McLaughlin and Olson (2017) with 63 transgender children and a matched sample of 53 cisgender children found that psychological outcomes were on par for both groups. The important part of this research is that the 63 transgender children were being raised by parents who affirmed their gender, thus demonstrating that parents who are affirming have a significant role to play in their children's wellbeing. Research by Simons et al. (2013) similarly found that amongst a sample of 66 transgender children, those whose parents were affirming reported higher life satisfaction and lower rates of poor mental health. Research by Travers, Bauer and Pyne (2012) with 84 transgender young people also found that the young people who were strongly supported by their parents reported greater life satisfaction and more positive mental health than those who were not supported. The box below explores in more detail how parents may come to a place of being supportive.

Case Study 4: Ecologies of Support

Between appointments Trudy had managed to reconnect with an old friend, whom she had learnt was transgender. This friend, Ben, was also a friend of Mark's, and Mark had been surprisingly accepting when Trudy shared the information about Ben being transgender. This lead to a meeting between Trudy, Mark, and Ben, where Mark sat and listened to Ben's journey with an open mind. The information that Ben shared went a long way to challenging some of the misconceptions that Mark had, even if he admitted that he still struggled to accept that genitalia doesn't determine gender. What he could see, however, was how happy Ben was in his life.

On the basis of this meeting, Trudy agreed to attend a session with Mark. In the session Mark reported that he was more open to listening to Drew in terms of gender, 'even if it wouldn't be my choice if I had one'. For Mark, the important turning point was not simply meeting with Ben, but it was hearing that Ben had lost contact with one of his parents who was not willing to affirm him. Mark felt sure that he would struggle with Drew in terms of gender for a long time, but he also knew that he didn't want to lose his child.

Beyond this evidence for the positive effects of affirmative parenting on transgender children, other research has critically examined how parents may actively resist cisgenderism in their parenting. A key example of this appears in the work of Pyne (2016), who interviewed 15 parents who were affirming of their transgender children. Pyne's findings demonstrate that affirming parents who are critical of cisgenderism actively resist normative accounts of parenting in multiple ways. First, they take seriously the injunction to be led by their children, rather than insisting that adults always know best. In terms of their children's gender, then, understanding and affirming their child's gender was a product of a relationship between parents and children that recognised that both held unique knowledges that deserved respect, rather than perpetuating forms of developmentalism wherein parental knowledge is privileged over that of children. Second, and relatedly, Pyne's participants resisted what he refers to as the 'sacralising' of professional knowledge. Rather than seeing clinicians, for example, as holding especially privileged knowledge about transgender children, Pyne's participants again valued their children's knowledge about their gender. For Pyne's participants, an explanation of their child's gender was not needed, hence recourse to biological essentialism via medical 'diagnosis' was eschewed. Finally, the parents interviewed by Pyne actively sought to challenge cisgenderism in the world around them, focusing their attentions on the pathology of public institutions that stigmatise transgender children, rather than searching for an aetiology of their child's gender.

In a similar way, and returning to Ryan's (2016) research summarised above, in addition to identifying a large group of 'gender expansive' mothers, Ryan also identified a smaller group of 'gender subversive' mothers. These were mothers who were critical of gender norms prior to having a transgender child, and who responded to learning that a child was transgender in ways that were critical of normative accounts of transgender children. Some of Ryan's gender subversive mothers were critical of mainstream representations of transgender children which emphasise children moving from one binary category to another. For some participants even materials specifically written for transgender children were normative in their depictions of gender expression. As one of Ryan's participants noted, most books for transgender children are written from "the perspective of a mortified parent who is getting over their shit and wants their kid to know...they still love them" (p. 88). Ryan's gender subversive mothers, by contrast, didn't have 'shit to get over' in terms of their children, but instead were focused on how normative gender ideologies restrict the gender expression of all children, and in particular their transgender children. The box below explores in more detail how parents may enlist the support of others to work through their own assumptions about gender.

> **Case Study 5: Ecologies of Support**
>
> At our next appointment Annika reported that she had made some significant gains in terms of her understanding of gender expression. This had come from two unexpected sources. First, Jake had approached his mother to speak about how she was processing the sessions with Lucy. Jake also expressed to Annika his own concerns that sometimes he felt that she limited who he could be as a person. Jake wasn't transgender, but he felt that sometimes Annika curtailed his interests because she was so invested in encouraging him to be a boy in particular ways. Due to our previous conversations Annika was open to this conversation with Jake, and it led her to reflect on many of the parenting decisions she had made in the past, which were often based on her own fears or worries, most of which were unrelated to her children and more about her own childhood.
>
> The second source of support that Annika had drawn on was watching documentaries made by transgender women. In the documentaries Annika had learnt about the struggles that many women had in being accepted by their families. What Annika took from this was that although she had been very affirming of Lucy from the onset, she had been less than affirming of how Lucy wanted to express her gender. It was clear to Annika that what Lucy needed was space to express herself, and for Annika to be guided by Lucy.

Whilst still constituting a relatively small part of the literature on parents of transgender children, research by Pyne (2016) and Ryan (2016) represents an important and I would suggest growing theme within the literature, namely a critical approach to parenting transgender children that refuses normative narratives of loss, narratives which largely serve to blame transgender children or at the very least suggest that they must account for their gender. In my own clinical practice too I see a growing number of parents who actively resist normative narratives of being transgender, and instead are critical advocates for the rights of transgender children in terms of a diversity of gender expressions. These parents don't come to see me to work through loss, indeed they don't speak about loss as a narrative at all. Rather, they ask for my help to advocate for their children, and to develop ways to speak critically about gender so as to challenge cisgenderism.

Concluding Thoughts

In a way in this chapter it might seem like I am wanting to argue that transgender children should have access to normative modes of gendered expression if they wish, but also should not be limited to these normative modes in order to be affirmed. Yet this apparent dilemma speaks to the heart of an affirming approach that seeks to be critical of normative developmental accounts. There is no one 'transgender truth' or correct 'transgender journey'. Every transgender child will find their own way to gender expression, and accordingly, every parent must be guided by their child's journey. Treating children as experts on their gender, as per an affirming approach, is about more than listening when a child says 'I am this gender'. It is about listening to how they experience their gender, how they wish to express it, and leaving space for that to change over time as the child grows and learns even more about themselves. This point about change is evident in the box below.

Case Study 4: Reinforcement and Resistance

Following our previous session, Trudy, Mark, Drew and I were finally able to meet to speak about gender. Mark had made a commitment to ceasing his controlling behaviours and the family had already spent some time together ahead of a planned return of Trudy and Drew to the family household. Drew was, nonetheless, cautious with Mark in the room, but slowly grew more confident in speaking about gender. Drew was clear that they didn't yet know how they might express their gender, or even how they might wish to define it, but what they knew for sure was that being a boy and doing so in stereotypical ways felt intensely uncomfortable for them. What they wanted was time and space to speak in more detail about how they experience their gender, and to do so without pressure or expectations from Trudy and Mark.

> Trudy commented that she had never heard Drew speak so clearly and eloquently, and Mark agreed that he was impressed with how confident Drew was in speaking during the session. I suggested that sometimes speaking is the hardest thing, especially when we might feel that other people don't want to listen. Drew affirmed that what they needed most was for Trudy and Mark to listen, even if they didn't always like what they heard. This seemed like an important step towards Drew being able to explore their gender and to do so without fear of reprisal.

In this chapter I have also compared and contrasted the literature on parents of transgender children so as to (1) highlight how the developmental literature may reinforce cisgenderist assumptions about the role of parents in terms of children's gender expression, and (2) challenge the assumption within much of the literature that negative narratives are the only ones possible with regards to parents of transgender children. This is not to naively suggest that all parents will be affirming. Certainly, and as Case Study 4 included in this chapter would suggest, this is not always the case. But my point in this chapter has nonetheless been to emphasise that rather than making our primary focus be the role of parents in terms of children's gender *development*, our focus as clinicians might more usefully be on how parents try to shape their children's gender *expression*. This distinction is important, and relates back to Chap. 2 and my arguments about gender development. Certainly, gender development does not occur in a vacuum, but it is also not something for which parents are the puppet masters. Children are agentic in coming to an understanding of how they experience their gender. What parents do, in response, will either open up or shut down how they express it. This has been a constant thread in the second case study in this chapter, as we can see in the final box below.

> **Case Study 5: Reinforcement and Resistance**
> At our next session Lucy informed me that she had taken the lead in identifying a range of books that depicted children of a diverse range of genders engaging in a diverse range of activities. She wanted to show her mum that other people too shared her view that she could be whatever kind of girl she wanted to be. She was pleasantly surprised, when she shared the books with Annika, that Annika had already been doing some work of her own,

> including watching documentaries. Annika told Lucy that she could see how her approach to gender expression had been limiting for both of her children.
> I had also shared with Annika the details of a parent network that she had subsequently joined, and learnt a great deal from other parents in the network who were raising transgender children. Many of the parents had emphasised that being a strong advocate for a child requires parents to have worked hard on unpacking their own assumptions about gender. Annika felt she had come a long way in her thinking, but also knew she needed to do more work. This included working on how she expressed her own gender, which she knew was influenced, at least in part, by the views of her own parents and her own upbringing.

In conclusion, working with parents of transgender children is as much about working on helping them to identify the best ways to affirm their child, as it is about working on helping them to identify the best ways to affirm themselves. This can include helping parents to unpack their own assumptions about gender. It can include supporting parents to resist the injunction to measure themselves against other parents, and in so doing trying to find ways to justify affirming their child. It can include helping parents to resist pathologising narratives about transgender children. But perhaps most of all it involves working with parents to listen to children. In societies where children are still expected often to be seen but not heard, listening is a key skill from which all parents can benefit.

References

American Psychiatric Association. (2013). *Diagnostic and statistical manual of mental disorders (DSM-5)*. Washington, DC: American Psychiatric Association.

Aramburu Alegría, C. (2018). Supporting families of transgender children/youth: Parents speak on their experiences, identity, and views. *International Journal of Transgenderism, 19*(2), 132–143.

Bartholomaeus, C., & Riggs, D. W. (2017). *Transgender people and education*. New York: Palgrave Macmillan.

Durwood, L., McLaughlin, K. A., & Olson, K. R. (2017). Mental health and self-worth in socially transitioned transgender youth. *Journal of the American Academy of Child & Adolescent Psychiatry, 56*(2), 116–123.

Gregor, C., Hingley-Jones, H., & Davidson, S. (2015). Understanding the experience of parents of pre-pubescent children with gender identity issues. *Child and Adolescent Social Work Journal, 32*(3), 237–246.

Kane, E. W. (2006). "No way my boys are going to be like that!": Parents' responses to children's gender nonconformity. *Gender and Society, 20*, 149–176.

Meadow, T. (2011). 'Deep down where the music plays': How parents account for childhood gender variance. *Sexualities, 14*(6), 725–747.

Meadow, T. (2018). *Trans kids: Being gendered in the twenty-first century*. California: University of California Press.

Norwood, K. (2013). Grieving gender: Trans-identities, transition, and ambiguous loss. *Communication Monographs, 80*(1), 24–45.

Owen Blakemore, J. E., Berenbaum, S. A., & Liben, L. S. (2009). *Gender development*. New York: Psychology Press.

Pyne, J. (2016). "Parenting is not a job… It's a relationship": Recognition and relational knowledge among parents of gender non-conforming children. *Journal of Progressive Human Services, 27*(1), 21–48.

Rahilly, E. P. (2015). The gender binary meets the gender-variant child: Parents' negotiations with childhood gender variance. *Gender & Society, 29*(3), 338–361.

Riggs, D. W., & Bartholomaeus, C. (2018a). Gaslighting in the context of clinical interactions with parents of transgender children. *Sexual and Relationship Therapy, 33*, 382–394.

Riggs, D. W., & Bartholomaeus, C. (2018b). Cisgenderism and certitude: Parents of transgender children negotiating educational contexts. *TSQ, 5*, 67–82.

Riggs, D. W., & Due, C. (2015). Support experiences and attitudes of parents of gender variant children. *Journal of Child and Family Studies, 24*(7), 1999–2007.

Rosen, W. D., Adamson, L. B., & Bakeman, R. (1992). An experimental investigation of infant social referencing: Mothers' messages and gender differences. *Developmental Psychology, 28*(6), 1172–1178.

Ryan, K. N. (2016). "My mom says some girls have penises": How mothers of gender-diverse youth are pushing gender ideology forward (and how they're not). *Social Sciences, 5*(4), 73–94.

Simons, L., Schrager, S. M., Clark, L. F., Belzer, M., & Olson, J. (2013). Parental support and mental health among transgender adolescents. *Journal of Adolescent Health, 53*(6), 791–793.

Travers, R., Bauer, G., & Pyne, J. (2012). *Impacts of strong parental support for trans youth: A report prepared for Children's Aid Society of Toronto and Delisle Youth Services*. Toronto: Trans Pulse.

Wren, B. (2002). 'I can accept my child is transsexual but if I ever see him in a dress I'll hit him': Dilemmas in parenting a transgendered adolescent. *Clinical Child Psychology and Psychiatry, 7*(3), 377–397.

5

Siblings, Grandparents, and Animal Companions

Of all the groups covered in this book, those covered in this chapter – siblings and other family members – are the most overlooked. To a certain degree this is surprising given that affirming approaches to working with transgender young people have increasingly recognised the importance of using systemic modalities, such as family therapy, in order to ensure that the lives of transgender children are understood holistically. At the same time, however, the lack of attention to family members beyond transgender children and their parents is not surprising. Given what we know of the pathologising history of mental health responses to transgender young people, it is not surprising that a primary focus on children and their parents has sat at the heart of pathologising approaches (where transgender young people are seen as problems to be solved, and where parents are seen as the cause of the problem, as we explored in Chap. 4).

As I will argue in this chapter, focusing on family members beyond parents is important for a number of reasons. First, it is important because transgender children and their parents do not exist in isolation from other family members. Second, and as the GENDER mnemonic emphasises, identifying ecologies of support is vital to affirming approaches, and such

© The Author(s) 2019
D. W. Riggs, *Working with Transgender Young People and their Families*, Critical and Applied Approaches in Sexuality, Gender and Identity,
https://doi.org/10.1007/978-3-030-14231-5_5

ecologies can often extend far beyond the parents and friends of transgender young people. Third, and just like parents as we explored in Chap. 4, other family members can be both a source of support, and a source of distress. Most family members (with one notable exception, as I will introduce below) are not exempt from the effects of cisgenderism. This may mean that other family members can witness cisgenderism and need the skills with which to respond, or other family members can enact cisgenderism. Together, it is for these three reasons that focusing on family members other than transgender young people and their parents is important when it comes to adopting an affirming approach. The box below outlines the beginnings of one case example where siblings and other family members were central to the experiences of one transgender young people.

> **Case Study 6: Gender Journey and Understanding**
> Hannah first came to see me at age nine, with her mothers Lisa and Kris. Lisa and Kris presented as entirely affirming of Hannah, citing their experience as lesbian women as key to their understanding of Hannah's needs. Hannah had first disclosed that she was transgender to her mothers when she was four, and the family had quickly agreed to facilitate Hannah's social transition ahead of starting school. Hannah has one older brother, Adam, who is two years older than Hannah.
> Hannah felt that she benefited from her mothers being open to a range of gender expressions. She was keenly aware of her mothers' own gender expressions as not being especially feminine, and stated that this had enabled her to explore her own ways of expressing herself as a girl. Hannah was also aware that her brother Adam was very non-conforming in his gender as male, however that was very different to her, as Adam was not transgender (or had not expressed this to date), but she was. This comparison was important to Hannah as it was one way that she signalled the truth of her gender (i.e., she was making a distinction between gender and expression).

In terms of the contents of this chapter, I follow previous chapters in weaving findings from developmental literature with a critical interpretation of such literature so as both to challenge their normative assumptions, whilst at the same time demonstrating how existing research may encompass transgender young people. I do this most clearly in the first section below, where I focus on cisgender siblings of transgender young people. In terms of siblings, I specifically focus on how cisgender siblings may often represent the nexus of cisgenderism and affirmation, and how we can work productively in this space. I then turn to consider the limited information on grandparents of transgender young people, and explore how, in different ways, grandparents too may sit at the nexus of cisgenderism and affirmation, and how their wisdom as grandparents may be harnessed in the service of the latter. In the final section of the chapter I consider the notable exception mentioned above, namely animal companions. Animals who live in the home and who are considered part of the family may have a special role to play in the lives of transgender young people. A focus on animal companions adds an extra dimension to clinical work that is all too often human-centric in its approach.

Siblings

In terms of the developmental literature on cisgender children, siblings are often seen as constituting a key form of influence upon both gender development and expression. Siblings can be both kith and kin. They are siblings and hence part of a family dynamic, but they are also peers, and may also be friends. Importantly, however, this is not to suggest that sibling relationships are absent of power. Age, birth order, and gender differences can often translate into opportunities for siblings to utilise such differences to their own advantage in the context of broader family dynamics. It is for this reason that I suggested in the introduction to this chapter, and as we shall explore in more detail below, that siblings of transgender young people can be both sources of strength, but also potential sources of distress.

In terms of the literature specifically, there is a tendency within the literature on siblings and gender to focus on siblings as in some way causative of outcomes for one another. This is evident in research that has focused on sibling relationships and homosexuality, and sibling relationships and enactments of masculinity and femininity. As Owen Blakemore, Berenbaum and Liben (2009) summarise, older siblings can influence the gender expression of younger siblings so that it more closely mirrors that of the older siblings. For example, children with older brothers tend to report themselves as more masculine, and to have more stereotypically masculine interests, than children who do not have older brothers. Notably, the same has not been found to be true for older sisters, who may introduce younger siblings to more stereotypically feminine interests, but research suggests that this does not fundamentally change the gender expression or interests of younger siblings.

Such research is problematic for a number of reasons. First, it treats masculinity and femininity as inherent to boys and girls respectively, thus making younger female siblings of older brothers, for example, a point of interest in regards to the influence of older brothers. That younger siblings might engage in gender expressions entirely of their own making is thus largely overwritten in the research on siblings and gender, thus minimising attention to the agency of younger siblings. In other words, to a degree the research on the influence of older siblings mistakes correlation for causation. Second, and similar to the research on homosexuality (which in the past suggested that the more older brothers a boy has the more likely he is to be gay), the literature on sibling influence on gender can inadvertently serve to provide an aetiology of being transgender. This is a problem as not only does it serve to warrant etiological accounts, but it also denies the agency of transgender young people in terms of them being the experts on their gender, independent of the 'influence' of others.

Conversely, the literature offers findings that may be considered useful with regard to transgender young people and their siblings. Specifically, and as Owen Blakemore, Berenbaum and Liben (2009) again summarise, whilst we know that in peer relationships gender stereotyping is the norm (and as we explored in Chap. 3, can negatively impact the capacity of transgender young people to express their gender), in sibling relationships it has been found that gender stereotyped play may be somewhat less prevalent. This is particularly true of siblings of different assumed genders, where both siblings are able to engage in a range of forms of play that are not limited to assumptions about their gender. For transgender young people exploring and coming to understand their gender, then, sibling relationships may offer the possibility of gaining insight as to how other people express their gender. For example, a transgender girl who has not yet disclosed that she is transgender, and who has a sister, may be supported and encouraged by her sister to explore her gender and engage in activities typically not available to her on the basis of her assigned sex.

The literature on sibling relationships also suggests that, different to both peer and parent-child relationships, sibling relationships can be premised more on enjoyment and share activities than on competition. This, however, is most certainly not uniformly true, and for transgender young people and their cisgender siblings it may be inflected in very specific ways. Ehrensaft (2011) suggests that assumptions about sibling relationships being less focused on competition can be especially untrue for transgender young people and their siblings. Cisgender siblings may feel that much of the family's attention and resources goes on the transgender sibling, and that they must compete for attention and resources. Conversely, transgender siblings may feel that, by comparison, their cisgender siblings 'have it easier', not having to negotiate cisgenderism and discrimination. The box below explores how Hannah experienced her relationship with her brother Adam.

Case Study 6: Expressed Concerns

In our second session, Hannah indicated that she had a concern she needed to speak about. In the first session, with her brother present, she had felt unable to inform us all that at times her brother misgendered her, and that she felt this was done on purpose. Lisa and Kris were quick to suggest that they had not witnessed any misgendering, and were surprised (and appeared to struggle to believe) that a child of theirs would intentionally misgender someone.

This lead to a second point of concern being raised by Hannah, namely that at times she felt that her mothers over emphasised their understanding of what it means to be transgender. As two cisgender women, Lisa and Kris felt a sense of solidarity with Hannah, and often referred to their own experiences as girls to respond to Hannah's feelings and experiences. Hannah stated that she was very thankful for her mothers and all they do to affirm her, but that she also felt that sometimes the fact that they are not transgender means that they overlook some of her experiences, or assume they are the same their own. This was especially true with regards to Adam. Hannah felt that her mothers were unable (or unwilling) to see instances of misgendering because they believed that (1) siblings are inherently supportive of one another and (2) that being raised in a lesbian household mitigates one having prejudicial views.

Ehrensaft (2011) suggests further areas where the sibling relationship may be inflected in specific ways for transgender young people and their cisgender siblings. Cisgender siblings may constitute a risk for transgender young people with regard to implicit or explicit threats to disclose that a child is transgender to people outside of the family due to "malice, power-mongering and sheer immaturity or spontaneity" (p. 170). The threat of disclosure adds a layer of complexity to sibling power relationships for transgender young people, who may feel compelled to keep a sibling onside, potentially at great costs to themselves in terms of self expression and resistance to sibling demands. Conversely, cisgender siblings can be useful points of differentiation for parents, and allow for leverage in decision making about transgender children when it comes to self expression. For example, a transgender girl who wishes to wear nail polish may state that refusing permission means her parents are being transphobic. An older female sibling who is also not allowed to wear nail polish due to the parents' own values is a useful comparison point, as it can serve to highlight to the transgender sibling that not wearing nail polish is a reflection of the parents' values about gender expression and age more broadly, rather than being transgender-specific.

For cisgender siblings too, there are specific inflections that can warrant clinical attention. As discussed in Chap. 3, the privacy versus secret distinction is an important one. This is a distinction that maintains that being transgender is private information to be shared at the discretion of the person, but it is not *per se* a secret. Yet at the same time, and as Ehrensaft (2011) discusses, how might a young cisgender sibling understanding this distinction: how might 'privacy' be seen as a negative, rather than positive characteristic, and what message might this give about being transgender? Further with regards to messages about being transgender, both Ehrensaft (2011) and Tando (2016) suggest that it is important not to assume that cisgender siblings will automatically 'get' what it means to be transgender. This signals the importance of active and purposive discussions with cisgender siblings about key concepts, such as pronouns and terminology. As is true for many cisgender people living in cisgenderist societies, being an ally is not a default position. Rather, it is one that must be actively learnt, and one that requires constant reflection: there is no perfect ally, given being an ally typically means that one is not transgender, and hence one does not have the same or similar lived experiences. I explore this point in more detail in the box below with regard to Hannah's brother Adam. Nonetheless, and as is indicated anecdotally, siblings are often the staunchest supporters of transgender young people, the suggestion being that siblings are more likely to already be aware of transgender people's lives, and to have more positive views than older generations (Fink and Scott 2015; Pullen Sansfaçon et al. 2015; Whyatt-Sames 2017).

> **Case Study 6: Necessary Actions**
> I asked Lisa and Kris if they could bring Adam to our next session. Adam came along, and was very willing to speak with me. He was very clear that Hannah is his sister, but also stated that sometimes he feels like his mothers favour Hannah: favour her because she is a girl, and favour her because she needs "extra things" (such as appointments with me). Adam admitted that whilst at first he accidentally used the wrong pronouns because it took him some time to make the cognitive switch, this was many years ago. The recent instances of misgendering, he admitted, were done on purpose to assert some sort of control in the family dynamic.
> Lisa and Kris were dismayed to hear that Adam had been misgendering Hannah on purpose. But they were also able to see that some of their assumptions about being an inclusive family had laid the groundwork for misgendering to become a tool for sibling control. Rather than equally focusing on Adam, or at least checking in with him to ensure he was okay, they had assumed that he was okay. Adam mentioned that he was very interested in attending karate classes, and Kris suggested that she was more than happy to take him weekly so that they could have some time together. We also discussed the possibility that Adam might join in with a group of other cisgender siblings who meet regularly. Adam was particularly taken by this idea as he liked the idea of making new friends who would understand his life, and also saw it as an opportunity to grow in his understanding of what it means to be an ally.

Finally with regard to siblings, it is important to recognise that siblings can be caught up in the nexus of love for a sibling and the wish to be a strong ally, and fears about being discriminated against themselves, as well as the costs that may come from parents encouraging (particularly older) siblings to 'look out for' a transgender sibling, especially at school. This is not for a moment to suggest that cisgender siblings have it harder than their transgender siblings. Rather, it is to suggest that, given the broader context of cisgenderism, *all* family members can be negatively affected, even if this is most acutely felt by transgender family members. Cisgender siblings can thus often need support to work through their own concerns and experiences, both to be happier within themselves, but also to be equipped to know how best to support a transgender sibling.

Grandparents

Turning to consider the grandparents of transgender young people, there are two competing narratives about grandparents that are likely as applicable to cisgender children as they are to transgender children. The first narrative is of the doting grandparent who, by default of being one step removed (i.e., not actively parenting a grandchild in most cases), can provide unconditional positive regard for a grandchild, and a refuge if needed from parents. The second narrative is one that emphasises grandparents as emblematic of older generations who have outdated views and are more likely to be set in their ways and unwilling to listen to children. I will now explore each of these in turn.

In terms of grandparents providing unconditional positive regard to grandchildren, some researchers have emphasised theories of 'kinkeeping', with grandmothers in particular viewed as invested in maintaining relationships across generations. This has been suggested as being especially true for grandmothers who have close relationships with their daughters and in turn also granddaughters (Attar-Schwartz et al. 2009). Yet some researchers have found that such gender normative assumptions may not always hold true. Grandfathers too might be focused on kinkeeping, and grandparents of any gender might share close relationships with grandchildren of any gender (Dubas 2001). Uniform across this research, however, is the finding that parents can often be gatekeepers to close intergenerational relationships.

For transgender young people, research findings about cisgender young people and their grandparents might in some instances be applicable. Specifically, the finding that in some families grandparents might enjoy close relationships with grandchildren regardless of gender suggests that it is the quality and characteristics of the relationship that are important, rather than gender. As such, a grandparent who shares a close relationship with a grandchild may be an important source of support if the child discloses that they are transgender. The literature on cisgender children and their grandparents also suggests that grandparents can play an important role when the parent-child relationship is in crisis or under stress (Owen Blakemore et al. 2009). Not to suggest for one moment that having a transgender child represents a 'crisis', but for some parents there can be stressors associated with a child disclosing that they are transgender, stressors that arise from the broader context of cisgenderism. Previously existing close relationships between grandparents and grandchildren can thus be a useful resource through the process of disclosure and adjustment.

Ehrensaft (2011) writes that she often receives emails from grandparents wanting to know how best to support a transgender grandchild. Ehrensaft suggests that it is grandparents' "wisdom of age" (p. 68), and the fact that they are typically not invested in parenting their grandchildren, which allows some grandparents to take a step back from their own assumptions and stereotypes to be supportive of a transgender grandchild. Yet as was true for cisgender siblings, for a cisgender grandparent to be an ally requires work: love is not enough. For some 'older old' grandparents, learning new terminology may be cognitively challenging, and remembering a change in pronouns or name may be difficult. This is not to reinforce ageist assumptions about older people, but rather to acknowledge the specific challenges that may present clinically in working with the extended family members of transgender young people. There may also be generational differences in how gender and family matters are spoken about. Some grandparents may not speak with their friends about a grandchild being transgender. This may have little to do with being embarrassed or ashamed, and more to do with generational beliefs about what information should or should not be shared. Conversations in the clinical context with transgender young people about this can often be important, as it provides an opportunity to highlight that grandparents can be proud and affirming without necessarily speaking about their grandchild's gender publicly (though some grandparents are indeed vocal public advocates).

Of course as noted in the opening to this section, there are at least two dominant narratives about grandparents. One, already canvassed above, pertains to the doting and caring grandparent. But we also know that for some transgender young people grandparents can be anything but this. Budge (2015), for example, reports on the narrative of a transgender young person whose grandfather in particular called her a 'freak', and was entirely unwilling to engage in respectful dialogue. Beyond this account and one provided by Ehrensaft (2011) of a step-grandfather shaming a transgender granddaughter, very little has been documented about grandparents who are less than accepting or who entirely reject a transgender grandchild. Nonetheless, it is reasonable to suggest that some grandparents will struggle, and may choose to remove themselves from their grandchild's life. This may compound the challenges already faced by some parents, and place transgender children in the middle. For some transgender young people who do not share a close relationship with their grandparents, they may be able to reconcile a grandparent's disengagement. For other young people, however, a grandparent who refuses to affirm them may constitute a significant loss arising from cisgenderism. As such, as clinicians we must be mindful of instances where a family member such as a grandparent chooses to distance themselves, and the need to work on this in the clinical context so as to support transgender young people through such losses. In the box below I explore the role of grandparents in Hannah's family.

Case Study 6: Distress Management

At our next session, Adam was again present, and reported that he had enjoyed attending the social gathering for cisgender siblings. He noted, however, that for many of the siblings grandparents were a key part of their life. This had led Adam and Hannah to question their mothers about the relative absence of their grandparents. Both Lisa and Kris disclosed that, in the past they had told the children that their grandparents were largely absent (other than the occasional birthday or Christmas card) because they lived interstate. And this was partially true. What was also true was that both sets of grandparents had struggled to come to terms with their daughters being lesbian, and upon learning that one of their grandchildren was transgender, their struggles were compounded.

Both Hannah and Adam reported that they felt distressed that they didn't know this information. Lisa and Kris stated that they had wanted to shield their children from any distress that might come from knowing about the views of their grandparents, but could now see that perhaps they had done as much harm as good. Rather than focusing on the world as being comprised of both supportive people and people who are less than supportive or indeed who actively discriminate, Lisa and Kris had worked hard to create a life where the children were largely sheltered from discrimination.

As we discussed, this had potentially done very little to prepare Hannah and Adam for what it can be like to live in a world shaped by cisgenderism and heterosexism. Lisa and Kris could acknowledge that they wouldn't always be able to protect their children, and that talking about family members as a source of discrimination was one way of introducing the topic. This led to robust conversations amongst the four about how they might reach out to the grandparents, both acknowledging their own views as older people, but also acknowledging their distress as children and grandparents at being alienated from some of their family.

Animals as Family Members

The field of human-animal studies has increasingly focused on humans who view animal companions who live in the home as family. Yet to date, relatively little research has focused specifically on children's views on animals as family. Morrow (1998) suggests a number of reasons as to why this might be the case. First, there is the historical conflation of animals and human children, such that both are seen as part of 'nature', not yet subject to or aware of the rules of human society (or in the case of animals, not privy to such rules by default of not being human). Such conflations are both developmentalist and anthropocentric: they position both animals and human children as second rate to human adults. Related to this, Morrow suggests a second point, namely that much of the research on animals and human children has focused on animals as sources of learning for child development. In this context animals are seen as objects through which human children learn about empathy and develop self-competencies. As a result, animals are not viewed as subjects with whom children may share kin relationships.

In Morrow's (1998) own research with nominally cisgender children, her participants described animals as more than simply objects, more than simply a testing ground for human child development. Instead, caring for animals was seen as part of a shared relationship between animals and children, one that was similar to shared relationships with humans. In terms of gender, Morrow suggests that the caring roles and relationships that her participants shared with animals were highly normative: girls were reported as nurturing and looking after animals, whereas boys were reported as playing with animals. Tipper's (2011) research with human children and their relationships with animals adds an extra dimension to the research of Morrow, highlighting the often very physical relationship that children of all genders share with animals, a physicality that may be largely absent from their relationships with other humans. It is this physicality, Tipper suggests, that may constitute animals as a very specific and much loved form of kin for human children.

Turning to consider transgender people specifically, research on the intersections of experiences of family violence and relationships with animal companions in the lives of transgender adults suggests that animals may be especially loved for the non-judgemental care they provide. Such research suggests that, in the face of cisgenderism and specifically discrimination and violence from family members, animal companions are seen by many transgender people as offering unconditional positive regard, and as providing a safe haven (Riggs et al. 2018; Taylor et al. 2018). With regard to transgender young people, the *From Blues to Rainbows* report noted that of the 189 young people surveyed, 63% stated that spending time with animals made them feel better (Smith et al. 2014), and in the *Trans Pathways* report 65.5% of the sample of 711 young people stated that they spent time with animals in order to feel better (Strauss et al. 2017). In the box below I explore how Hannah introduced an animal companion to our sessions.

Case Study 6: Ecologies of Support

In a follow up session Hannah proudly reported that she had found a way that she would go about writing to her grandparents. Hannah enjoyed a very close relationship with Molly, a dog who lived in the family home. For Hannah, Molly was like the sister she never had, with whom she shared many confidences, and who was the first person she spoke to about being transgender. As the years had passed and Molly had aged, Hannah was still very glad for their close relationship, and the degree of understanding and acceptance that she felt Molly showed towards her.

> Hannah suggested that she would write to her grandparents, using Molly as an example of what it can look like to be accepting. She had found photos of herself and Molly together, from a young age until the present, and planned to map out how Molly had remained the same caring cheery sibling to Hannah that she had always been. She thought this might show her grandparents that they too could be accepting and understanding. Hannah was also pragmatic: She noted that 'everyone loves dogs', and she felt that her grandparents, two of whom lived on a farm, might respond positively to photos of Molly.

In other research transgender young people have reported that animals are seen as an important gauge of relationships with other humans. For example, Jin (2018) reports that some transgender young people may first disclose their gender to an animal companion, and may later see an animal companion as a good judge of character when it comes to new human friends or intimate partners. Dietert and Dentice (2013) further suggest that for some transgender young people animals may be viewed as a marker of their gender. For example, Dietert and Dentice suggest that the young transgender boy they spoke with viewed his interest in 'unusual animals' (i.e., spiders and snakes) as a marker of his masculinity. Whilst we might want to be critical of such gender stereotypes, they nonetheless signal how relationships with animal companions can bring meaning to transgender young people's accounts of their gender.

Of course in many ways the examples provided above run afoul of the types of instrumentalisation that Morrow (1998) critiqued with regard to the literature on human children and animals. It is thus important that when we discuss animal companions with transgender young people we explore how they experience their *relationships* with animals. This might include asking about animals when compiling family genograms, and if it is clear that animals comprise a considerable source of meaning in a young person's life, that we enquire about this in detail, moving beyond instrumental benefits so as to encompass loving, reciprocal relationships between transgender young people and animals. Given the focus of the GENDER mnemonic on ecologies of support, it is vital to consider how animals may constitute a key form of support as kin, rather than as objects that function to mitigate cisgenderism. In other words, it would certainly seem to be the case from the limited previous literature that animals *do* function to mitigate cisgenderism, but they are more than that: they are sentient beings in their own rights with whom many transgender young people share meaningful relationships.

Finally in terms of animal companions, it is vital that we recognise that in being in relationships with humans, animals are placed at risk of violence directed towards humans. The literature has long pointed towards 'the link' between human-directed and animal-directed violence (Taylor et al. 2018). Meadow (2018) shares the story of one family who lived in a small town in the United States, a town that strongly opposed the mother's affirming approach to her transgender daughter. The family were forced to flee the town in fear of their lives, but sadly left an animal companion behind. The animal was later found murdered as retribution against the mother and daughter. Reading this story in a book full of powerful and moving stories, I am still left with an incredible sadness about how the animal must have suffered: the cost to them of cisgenderism and loving their human companions. None of this is to suggest, of course, that animal companions are at such risk when living with transgender people that they should be prevented from doing so: the risk lies with cisgenderism, not transgender people. But in celebrating the meaningful relationships that transgender people and animal companions share, we must always be mindful of the costs and risks as well as the joys to all parties.

Concluding Thoughts

In this chapter I have sought to move away from the almost exclusive focus on transgender young people and their parents in previous literature, to also encompass family relationships with siblings, grandparents, and animal companions. My intent in doing so was simple: many children live with siblings, many have at least one living grandparent and with whom they share a close relationship, and many live with animal companions. For transgender young people, then, it is important that we attend to the many differing kin relationships they experience, both those that bring joy and meaning, and those that potentially bring challenges and distress. In the final box below I focus on both joy and challenges as faced by Hannah and her family.

> **Case Study 6: Reinforcement and Resistance**
> A few sessions later, Hannah reported that she had some success with one set of grandparents. They had responded positively to her letter, and spoke positively about one day meeting Molly and the rest of the family. Hannah, Lisa, Kris and I then spoke about what types of information they might share with these grandparents ahead of a potential meeting, so that they had a better understanding about appropriate terminology. I reinforced to the family that setting their own ground rules was important, and that even if things didn't go entirely smoothly on their first meeting, they had options: to step back from the relationship again, or try a different approach to engaging the grandparents.
> Sadly, the other set of grandparents had declined to engage. They had returned Hannah's letter unopened. Following our previous conversations about the grandparents, and subsequent conversations within the family that were open and frank, both Hannah and Adam felt okay with the lack of response from this set of grandparents. They understood that not everyone in the world will be accepting, and that perhaps in some ways it is better to know this, rather than trying to force a relationship that could have been distressing for all. Hannah in particular noted again her love for Molly, and that she 'more than made up' for not having a relationship with her grandparents. Resisting the assumption that only humans can be kin, Hannah proudly claimed Molly as her sister.

When it comes to gender, and as I have outlined in this chapter, sibling relationships may be an important testing ground for transgender young people coming to understand and disclose their gender, just as sibling relationships may be particularly testing for transgender young people in terms of potential bullying or threats of disclosure. Working holistically with siblings can thus be an important opportunity for facilitating caring and supportive relationships for transgender young people. With regard to grandparents, it is reasonable to assume that for some transgender young people caring and close relationships with grandparents may continue, whilst for some young people grandparents may struggle to understand or be affirming. Including grandparents, even if primarily through discussions with parents, offers opportunities for identifying barriers to support, or conversely additional forms of support to supplement that provided by parents. It can also give parents an opportunity to speak about the challenges they may experience arising from their own parents' responses to a child being transgender. As I discussed in Chap. 4, challenging narratives of 'loss' amongst parents doesn't mean that as clinicians we should eschew talking about the very real losses that some families experience due to cisgenderism (i.e., a grandparent who disengages from the families because of their views on transgender people). Finally, recognising animal companions as kin offers an extra dimension to understanding how transgender young people create meaning in their lives. I certainly have worked with young people who have brought animals to sessions, and through whom we have at first communicated and developed rapport. Showing care for animals as a clinician can signal to children that you understand and value the relationships they share with animal companions (Zilcha-Mano et al. 2011). In sum, family members are an important part of the process of gender transition for many young people. They can be barriers to an affirming approach, or they can be the greatest of allies. Clinicians have a significant role to play in acknowledging the relationships that transgender young people share with a wide variety of kin, and to including where possible family in clinical work so as to facilitate the best outcomes for young people.

References

Attar-Schwartz, S., Tan, J. P., & Buchanan, A. (2009). Adolescents' perspectives on relationships with grandparents: The contribution of adolescent, grandparent, and parent–grandparent relationship variables. *Children and Youth Services Review, 31*(9), 1057–1066.
Budge, S. L. (2015). Psychotherapists as gatekeepers: An evidence-based case study highlighting the role and process of letter writing for transgender clients. *Psychotherapy, 52*(3), 287–297.
Dietert, M., & Dentice, D. (2013). Growing up trans: Socialization and the gender binary. *Journal of GLBT Family Studies, 9*(1), 24–42.
Dubas, J. S. (2001). How gender moderates the grandparent-grandchild relationship: A comparison of kin-keeper and kin-selector theories. *Journal of Family Issues, 22*(4), 478–492.
Ehrensaft, D. (2011). *Gender born, gender made: Raising healthy gender-nonconforming children.* New York: The Experiment.
Fink, M., & Scott, M. (2015). *OMG I'm trans.* Melbourne: Minus18.

Jin, J. N. (2018). *The clinical significant of companion animals for LGBT+ youth: Unconditional love in a straight society.* Unpublished PhD thesis, University of Pennsylvania.

Meadow, T. (2018). *Trans kids: Being gendered in the twenty-first century.* Oakland: University of California Press.

Morrow, V. (1998). My animals and other family: Children's perspectives on their relationships with companion animals. *Anthrozoös, 11*(4), 218–226.

Owen Blakemore, J. E., Berenbaum, S. A., & Liben, L. S. (2009). *Gender development.* New York: Psychology Press.

Pullen Sansfaçon, A., Robichaud, M. J., & Dumais-Michaud, A. A. (2015). The experience of parents who support their children's gender variance. *Journal of LGBT Youth, 12*(1), 39–63.

Riggs, D. W., Taylor, N., Signal, T., Fraser, H., & Donovan, C. (2018). People of diverse genders and/or sexualities and their animal companions: Experiences of family violence in a bi-national sample. *Journal of Family Issues, 39*, 4226–4247.

Smith, E., Jones, T., Ward, R., Dixon, J., Mitchell, A., & Hillier, L. (2014). *From blues to rainbows: The mental health and well-being of gender diverse and transgender young people in Australia.* Melbourne: Australian Research Centre in Sex, Health and Society (ARCSHS), La Trobe University.

Strauss, P., Cook, A., Winter, S., Watson, V., Wright Toussaint, D., & Lin, A. (2017). *Trans pathways: The mental health experiences and care pathways of trans young people.* Telethon Kids Institute, Perth.

Tando, D. (2016). *The conscious parent's guide to gender identity.* Avon: Adams Media.

Taylor, N., Riggs, D. W., Donovan, C., Signal, T., & Fraser, H. (Online First, 2018). People of diverse genders and/or sexualities caring for and protecting animal companions in the context of domestic violence. *Violence Against Women.* https://doi.org/10.1177/1077801218809942.

Tipper, B. (2011). 'A dog who I know quite well': Everyday relationships between children and animals. *Children's Geographies, 9*(2), 145–165.

Whyatt-Sames, J. (2017). Being brave: Negotiating the path of social transition with a transgender child in foster care. *Journal of GLBT Family Studies, 13*(4), 309–332.

Zilcha-Mano, S., Mikulincer, M., & Shaver, P. R. (2011). Pet in the therapy room: An attachment perspective on animal-assisted therapy. *Attachment & Human Development, 13*(6), 541–561.

6

Conclusion

Introduction

Throughout this book I have woven together an affirming approach to working with transgender young people and their families with a critical developmental approach to gender. This has consistently been a difficult task, given by default any developmental account runs the risk of slipping into developmentalism. My approach in this book, in order to mitigate the risk, has been to acknowledge that although the needs of transgender young people and their families change over time, there is no inherent normative order to such change. Whilst to a certain extent the case studies I have presented in this book follow a linear narrative in terms of sessions with clients, the issues that are presented do not necessarily map out a linear progression. In other words, simply because one part of the GENDER mnemonic comes later in the word order (i.e., ecologies of support comes after expressed concerns), this does not mean that cases must be formulated in a pre-determined order. At a first session support may be a key issue, and only in later sessions may discussions about gender journeys and understandings occur. Given case formulations are

© The Author(s) 2019
D. W. Riggs, *Working with Transgender Young People and their Families*, Critical and Applied Approaches in Sexuality, Gender and Identity,
https://doi.org/10.1007/978-3-030-14231-5_6

dynamic and flexible, the GENDER mnemonic offers a non-normative, non-linear approach to understanding development.

Throughout this book I have also paid central attention to the effects of cisgenderism. My attention to cisgenderism across all chapters in this book intersects with my critical developmental focus, providing an account of an affirming approach to working with transgender young people and their families that I believe to be relatively unique. This is not to say that other affirming approaches are not critical of social norms or do not focus on developmental issues. Rather, it is to suggest that in this book the interweaving of cisgenderism and development, with the former placed at the fore, has allowed me to create a space from which to consider many of the challenges that transgender young people and their families experience without positioning young people or their families as the locus of responsibility or as having to follow a specific developmental pathway. Importantly, my point here is not to deny the agency of young people and their families. Rather, it is to situate them within a broader context of cisgenderism, one that produces many of the challenges clinicians are likely to see. Narratives of loss on the part of parents, for example, or accounts of dysphoria by young people, are not inherent to either group. Rather, they are a product of cisgenderism. Acknowledging this, I would suggest, and making it central to this book, has allowed me to outline a critical developmental approach that resists a one size fits all model.

With the above points in mind in terms of the approach I have outlined in this book, in the sections that follow I examine a range of issues that extend upon the other chapters in this book with regard to my approach to working with transgender young people and their families. I first consider key barriers to affirming approaches and some of the ways in these barriers might be addressed. I then examine how I have used the GENDER mnemonic in training, and how clinicians who have undertaken training with me experience this particular approach to case formulation, and its role in increasing competency. Taking up the point above about non-linear approaches, I then highlight the importance of attending to ongoing changes in the care of transgender young people and their families, focusing on what currently constitute my taken for granted assumptions about best practice, but also highlighting where this is likely to change and what might drive such change. Returning to the opening chapter of this book, I then focus on how clinicians working across a range of disciplines can productively work together, despite potentially differing views on 'science' and 'gender'. Finally, I outline some of the areas that I believe warrant close attention in the future with regard to working with transgender young people and their families.

Barriers to Affirming Care

In terms of barriers to affirming care, it is arguably the case that all such barriers are the product of cisgenderism. As I will outline in this section, some barriers are a product of what, following Braun (2000) in her work on heterosexism in research, we might call cisgenderism by both commission and omission. Braun suggests that heterosexism by commission is constituted by explicit acts of heterosexism. In the case of barriers to affirming care, cisgenderism by commission might involve explicit biases on the part of clinicians that fail to show due care for transgender young people and their families, or explicit failures to be affirming (such as in clinic documentation or reports). In her work on heterosexism in research Braun also refers to heterosexism by omission, which is constituted by a failure to challenge heterosexism when it occurs. In terms of cisgenderism by omission, this may occur when clinicians privilege parent views over those of children, thus meaning that misgendering, for example, is left unchallenged. Cisgenderism by omission can also occur when as clinicians we fail to challenge one another's cisgenderism by commission.

Across the literature, cisgenderism by commission is the most common form of cisgenderism reported in terms of barriers to affirming care for young people. For example, in their study of parents of transgender children, Pullen Sansfaçon, Robichaud and Dumais-Michaud (2015) report that some parents experienced challenges when clinic documentation only included two gender options, or when assigned sex was recorded and used by staff instead of a child's gender. Gridley et al. (2016), in their interviews with transgender young people and their parents, reported misgendering to be a common experience, and for many this continued despite being corrected by young people and parents. Other forms of cisgenderism by commission identified by Gridley and colleagues included clinicians gatekeeping access to services (and in particular making young people wait for services unnecessarily, particularly with regard to puberty suppression), clinicians having no understanding of non-binary genders, and clinicians who insisted upon intensive therapy before considering any treatment (which is in direct contradiction to the World Professional Association for Transgender Health *Standards of Care* 2011).

Research conducted with transgender and gender diverse young people in the Australian context by Smith et al. (2014) has also identified instances of cisgenderism by commission. These included young people not being listened to or having their views discounted due to their age, clinicians making normative assumptions about gender expression (including encouraging or insisting upon stereotypical gendered interests and activities as an indicator that a young person is transgender), and clinicians sharing personal information about a young person's gender with other staff and the young person's parents without consent. Research by Pullen Sansfaçon et al. (2018) with transgender young people also reports on cisgenderism by commission in the form of what has been termed 'trans broken arm syndrome'. This refers to when a transgender person presents for emergency services, and when the person discloses that they are transgender, the treating professional focuses solely on their gender, and not on the actual presenting issue. For some of the young people in the study by Pullen Sansfaçon and colleagues, presenting for acute psychiatric care resulted in clinicians ignoring the actual mental health concern, and instead asking unnecessary and inappropriate questions about bodies and identities (see also Riggs and Bartholomaeus 2017).

Cisgenderism by commission may be the product of both ignorance and personal bias: it may be a product of a lack of experience or training, but it may also reflect the beliefs of individual clinicians with regard to transgender people. Given the predominance of so-called 'curative' (i.e., non-affirming) approaches to working with transgender young people up until very recently (and indeed in some places such approaches still predominate), it is perhaps unsurprising that approaches that are pathologising or which at the very least are dismissive of young people's views would be the most common. Yet a lack of awareness about current best practice approaches (i.e., those that are affirming) is different to clinicians holding negative views about transgender people. Whilst in previous research mental health clinicians have on average been found to hold positive views about transgender people, an average is simply that: it encompasses both those with very positive and informed views, and those with negative and uninformed views. In particular, research suggests that clinicians who are male, who are more religious, who are more politically conservative, and who are more wedded to normative gender ideologies are the most likely to engage in cisgenderism by commission (Brown et al. 2018; Riggs and Sion 2017).

In terms of cisgenderism by omission, this is arguably somewhat harder to identify, given doing so is either reliant upon naturalistic data involving discussions between clinicians (Braun used focus group data to identify heterosexism by omission), or requires clinicians to speak openly about their failures to challenge cisgenderism. Nonetheless, we can certainly point towards likely instances of cisgenderism by omission. These might include clinicians working with transgender young people and their families without having undertaken adequate training. Given that so many areas of mental health care require specialization, it would constitute a failure if clinicians worked with transgender young people and their families without sufficient knowledge. This is not to naively resort to the standard scientist-practitioner model in order to argue that only particular forms of evidence based practice are legitimate. Rather, it is to acknowledge that the literature summarised above clearly identifies (what may at times be purposive) forms of cisgenderism on the part of clinicians, and that awareness of this would indicate that being knowledgeable and informed is important so as to avoid cisgenderism by commission. Doing otherwise would thus constitute a form of cisgenderism by omission.

Cisgenderism by omission also occurs when clinicians hear terminology used that is widely recognised as problematic, and don't challenge it. Referring, for example, to a child as a 'natal male', or to someone's 'birth sex', are forms of problematic terminology. Hearing these used by other clinicians and not challenging them is a form of cisgenderism by omission. Thinking back to Chap. 4, and the ways in which some parents may speak about or seek to manage their children's gender expression, we might also suggest that failing to challenge this in the clinical space could constitute a form of cisgenderism by omission. Certainly I make it clear to the parents that I work with that I will always politely correct misgendering: to do otherwise would be cisgenderism by omission on my part. More broadly I also focus on challenging normative assumptions about gender expression, including when parents might draw on stereotypes about what children of a particular gender should or should not do.

In terms of addressing both cisgenderism by commission and omission, young people in previous research have clearly elaborated how the former may be addressed. This includes clinicians being trained in gender affirming approaches, not using outdated terminology, not being judgmental or hostile, and not misgendering (Gridley et al. 2016). For both cisgenderism by commission and omission, training is thus vital. Such training should explicitly address cisgenderism as a concept, outline affirming approaches (including diversity in gender expression, rather than focusing solely on gender binaries), address relevant professional society guidelines, and include a focus on personal biases and assumptions (Riggs and Bartholomaeus 2016). Also important for addressing cisgenderism by commission and omission is clinical supervision. Whilst research shows that experience working with transgender young people results in increased competency (Riggs and Bartholomaeus 2016), it should not be the job of young people and their families to educate clinicians. Undertaking ongoing supervision so as to identify potential instances of cisgenderism in practice is an important way to avoid cisgenderism by omission.

Efficacy of the GENDER Mnemonic

Having utilised the GENDER mnemonic throughout this book, I felt it important to share how I have sought to ascertain its utility to other clinicians. I do this not to provide an 'evidence base' for the mnemonic *per* se, but rather to show how other clinicians I have undertaken training with have responded to it as a means to case formulation. In terms of training, and since developing the GENDER mnemonic, I have been fortunate to have many opportunities to use it in events that I have run for mental health clinicians. Informal feedback has consistently indicated that clinicians find the mnemonic intuitive to use, and a useful guide for directing sessions with transgender young people and their families. To formally assess the GENDER mnemonic in training, in 2018 I ran a series of four webinars for the Australian Psychological Society, focused on affirming approaches to working with transgender young people and their families. The series provided information to attendees about the GENDER mnemonic, and attendees had the opportunity to apply it to a series of case studies. Of the 85 attendees, 50 consented to participate in a study that involved completing a questionnaire prior to the first webinar, and another after completing the webinar series. Both questionnaires included a measure of confidence in working clinically with transgender young people, a measure of comfort in working clinically with transgender young people, and a series of open-ended questions asking participants to describe their understandings of 'cisgenderism', 'transgender', and 'non-binary' gender. The second questionnaire also included open-ended questions about the GENDER mnemonic, and other questions related to learning derived from the webinar series.

Comparing responses from webinar participants it was clear that taking part in the series increased both confidence and comfort. Both were measured on a five-point scale. Prior to participating in the webinar series, the average score for comfort was 2.5, meaning that on average participants were somewhat comfortable in working with transgender young people. Following the webinar series, the average score for comfort was 4.7, meaning that on average participants were almost very comfortable in working with transgender young people. Similarly for confidence, prior to participating in the webinar series the average score for confidence was 2.1, meaning that on average participants did not feel confident in working with transgender young people. Following the webinar series, the average score for confidence was 4.6, meaning that on average participants were almost very confident in working with transgender young people.

In terms of understanding of key terms, prior to the webinar series the majority of participants could not define 'cisgenderism', and those who could provide responses such as 'it is a form of discrimination', or 'the idea that gender should match sex'. Following the webinar series participants, almost uniformly, could recount the definition of cisgenderism outlined in the introduction to this book. With regard to the terms 'transgender' and 'non-binary', prior to the webinar series most descriptions provided about the former used words such as 'match' or 'align' (i.e., 'someone whose gender does not align with their sex'). The webinar series addressed the point that both words are themselves forms of cisgenderism (i.e., gender is only seen as normatively 'matching' assigned sex because of cisgenderism). Prior to the webinar series the majority of participants could not provide a definition of 'non-binary', though those who did often treated transgender and non-binary as synonymous. Following the webinar series, which provided definitions for both terms, participants almost uniformly could describe both terms in ways that were mindful of cisgenderism and normative gender binaries.

When asked about what they most enjoyed about the webinar series, a repeated comment was the strength of the application of the GENDER mnemonic to clinical case studies, and the opportunity to work through the case studies using the mnemonic. In terms of the mnemonic itself, participants provided comments such as 'it is already helping to guide my work', 'I have shared it with other clinicians in my team who find it a really useful tool', and 'having a guide helps me feel more confident when this area is so complex and there is so much information to understand'. Informal comments about the GENDER mnemonic from other training events that I have run include 'as a psychologist who sees case formulation rather than diagnosis to be my core business, the mnemonic is vital to my work', and 'I can't help but feel that being exposed to something like the mnemonic sooner in my work with transgender young people would have greatly increased my competency – but glad to have it now'.

Of course the astute reader may question, given my critique of science outlined in the first chapter of this book, why I would undertake an assessment of the webinar series and report it here. Certainly, reporting change across time in terms of confidence and comfort (both of which were statistically significant) is normatively mired in a received understanding of science, where statistical significance accords weight to fact claims. This information, however, is only included for the interested reader who finds between-groups research interesting, and who is mindful of their limitations. For me, the interesting material appears in open-ended responses included above. To me these indicate that clinicians, most of whom were trained in the scientist-practitioner model, are open to incorporating critical thinking into their work, and that critical approaches to understanding working with transgender young people and their families offer a significant intervention into cisgenderism. Having a clear understanding of cisgenderism and being able to apply it in practice potentially means that clinicians will be mindful of their own biases and those of their colleagues. Furthermore, that the mnemonic was so well received indicates to me that it is a useful way to engage in case formulation in ways that are non-normative and non-linear.

Of course, as with any clinical tool, it will be interesting to see how it is engaged with, developed, and assessed into the future. One particular application that I think it lends itself well to is to clinicians ourselves. It is vital that we reflect on our own gender journeys and understandings, including our biases. It is important that we identify our own concerns when it comes to particular cases. Such concerns may result in necessary actions, such as consulting with colleagues, as I will explore in more detail below. For some of us, witnessing a child not being affirmed can be distressing, and more broadly, it is likely that for many of us there will be times when an affirming approach comes under attack from those who seek to pathologise transgender people's lives. This too can be distressing. Just like young people and their families, we need to adopt an ecological approach to support, identifying a broad range of people to whom we can turn, and this can involve providing reinforcement to *ourselves* that the work we are doing is just. This can occur alongside working to reinforce our colleagues and they us in return, and creating opportunities for resistance, a topic I will return to at the close of this chapter.

Shifting Practice Contexts

Clinicians working with transgender young people and their families do so in the context of multiple factors shaped by cisgenderism. Professional societies are for the most part now strong advocates for affirming approaches, however what constitutes 'affirming' may still be tempered by relative awareness of cisgenderism and how it shapes the language used. Terms such as 'match' or 'align', as described above, are still evident in the policies of some professional organisations. This gives somewhat unclear messages about how best to approach issues of terminology. The media is another key context in which clinicians practice. In the United Kingdom at present, for example, a negative focus on transgender young people dominates the tabloid news media. Discussions about so-called 'rapid onset gender dysphoria', as I addressed in Chap. 2, are used to discredit those who adopt affirming approaches, and indeed to discredit transgender young people and their families. Whilst clinical approaches should not be influenced by negative media, it is nonetheless important that clinicians are mindful of how such external forces shape the experiences of transgender young people and their families, and thus the importance of clinical authority in speaking out against negative messages.

Schools are another key context where contestations over transgender young people's lives occur (Bartholomaeus and Riggs 2017). In countries such as Australia, the United Kingdom, and the United States affirming approaches in schools appear to be applied piecemeal, which can create uncertainty for transgender young people and their families. As documented by Meadow (2018), schools can be a key site where young people and their parents are regulated, including parents being reported to child protective services for 'abusing a child' (when in fact what they are doing is affirming a child). Again, clinicians have an important role to play in engaging with schools so as to provide education, though I would also note that clinicians working in schools also need to ensure that they are sufficiently trained and skilled for working with transgender young people (Riggs and Bartholomaeus 2015).

Given the likelihood that negative messages about transgender young people and their families will persist, at least for the moment, it is important that clinicians are aware of and are able to clearly stake out a claim to knowledge. This is not to reify clinical knowledge *per se*, but rather to have critical literacy about why we do the work we do. Guidelines such as those contained in the Royal Children's Hospital in Melbourne, Australia, are internationally recognised as leading the way in terms of outlining affirming approaches (see Telfer et al. 2017). For myself, the things I take for granted are as follows. Young people are the experts on their gender. Young people do not *need* therapy in regards to their gender, though may benefit from support and opportunities to talk through their desires and needs, as well as in terms of distress arising from cisgenderism (a point I take up in more detail below). Clinicians do not need to diagnose gender dysphoria, though we do need to understand if young people experience it, and we need to be able to account for the work we do with young people and their families. Clinicians should not delay providing young people access to puberty blockers – there is absolutely no evidence to suggest that children are benefited by experiencing the puberty associated with their assigned sex. Young people have the right to conversations about fertility preservation, though should not be pressured into fertility preservation, particularly if such pressure reflects the desires of parents (i.e., for grandchildren). There is no predetermined age at which young people should commence hormone therapies, though ideally transgender young people should not be required to wait to commence such therapies until they are of a particular age. Lengthy periods on puberty blockers are contraindicated, and not being able to experience the puberty associated with one's along with one's peers can cause significant distress.

Importantly, the above points likely in places represent a shift in my thinking from a decade ago, and will likely shift again in the future. This is at least partly because, as more young people are affirmed at younger ages, their experiences are likely to be quite different to people from previous generations. For example, and as we saw in Chap. 3, puberty blockers may, for some young people, minimise dysphoria, but then other issues may arise in terms of how to talk about and negotiate with puberty in terms of peers. Similarly, in the past fertility preservation was often not considered, with infertility a presumed (and in some contexts prescribed) outcome of gender transition. Now that the reproductive rights of transgender people are increasingly recognised, this brings with it the need to have conversations with young people that we likely were not having in the past. Asking 'might you want to have children in the future?' of a 10 year old without resorting to developmentalism is, however, likely a difficult question to answer. Certainly, some young people and their parents may choose fertility preservation 'just in case', however I have argued elsewhere that 'just in case' is not an approach that clinicians should necessarily advocate for (Riggs 2019; Riggs and Bartholomaeus 2018a). We do not want to get caught up in pronatalist assumptions in our work, just as we don't want to undermine the reproductive rights of transgender young people. What we need to engage in are sensitive and thoughtful conversations about the future that start with a range of options, rather than simplistically endorsing fertility preservation for young people.

Facilitating Linked Up Care

Ensuring that clinical practice with transgender young people and their families is capable of staying abreast of current contexts and shifting clinical needs requires a linked up approach to care provision. Depending on the country, healthcare system, and epistemic weight given to differing professions, clinical practice with transgender young people and their families will be led by a range of professional groups. This will also be differentiated by the age of the young person. For example, very young children may require little interaction with medical professionals, however this likely shifts as children age and they require, for example, support from endocrinologists. Linked up care requires that rather than working in silos or privileging one particular profession, all clinicians work in partnership in order to meet the needs of young people and their families.

A key challenge to linked up care is the differing views that professions may have on 'science' and 'gender'. As I explored in the first chapter of this book, the meaning of science will depend on training, and the weight given to particular approaches to both research and what is construed as evidence-based practice. Medical practitioners, for example, may privilege clinical trials, whereas clinical social workers may privilege the views of clients developed in partnership with clinicians and researchers. Each of these approaches have their merits, though it is important to be mindful of how, historically, medical approaches have dominated the field of transgender healthcare, often to the detriment of transgender people. The same is true for understandings of gender. Most of the mental health professions have historically conflated gender with assigned sex, as I outlined in the first chapter of this book. Whilst there has been a slow shift in this regard, remnants of this are still evident when we see terms such as 'birth sex' or 'natal female' are used. Thinking in more complex and critical ways about gender requires clinicians to engage in cross disciplinary discussions. Mental health disciplines, for example, have a lot to gain from engagement with scholars and practitioners of gender studies, sociology, and cultural studies. And of course clinicians have much to learn from transgender communities. This is not to say that transgender people should have to educate clinicians. Rather, it is to highlight the importance of community engagement.

Returning to the topic of cisgenderism by omission, it is important never to underestimate the value of supervision or peer discussions. These can be important opportunities for growth in terms of clinical skills. They can also be vital opportunities to map out aspects of the GENDER mnemonic. In an article on gaslighting by parents of transgender young people (Riggs and Bartholomaeus 2018b), I explored how multidisciplinary conversations about shared cases allowed me to identify instances of gaslighting, and to develop with colleagues a unified approach. Working in isolation can at times be a barrier to action if as individual clinicians we are unsure about what we are seeing. Peer discussions offer opportunities to work through potential barriers or challenges, and to implement strategies across clinical teams for addressing them.

Areas Requiring Further Attention

As I noted in the introduction to this book, my focus primarily has been on transgender young people who have a binary gender. This has not been intended to be exclusionary of non-binary or agender young people, for example, but rather to recognise their specific needs that warrant focused attention. Certainly recent research suggests, for example, that non-binary young people as compared to transgender young people who have a binary gender are more likely to experience barriers to accessing medical services (e.g., hormones) (Clark et al. 2018). Only recently a colleague asked me why non-binary young people want to access services at all. Through discussion, it became evident that this colleague understood 'non-binary' to mean 'no gender at all', the assumption then being that non-binary young people would not wish to start puberty blockers or hormone therapies (i.e., that they would not wish to gender their body in a particular way). Whilst for some non-binary young people this may be true, the assumption that it will be true for all represents a barrier to affirming care for non-binary young people.

Another recent study reported that non-binary young people experience higher rates of anxiety and depression than transgender young people who have a binary gender (Thorne et al. 2018). The researchers suggest that this may be because of a relative lack of understanding of non-binary genders in most sectors of society, such that non-binary young people experience a considerable and ongoing burden to account for themselves. In the section above on barriers to care I touched on clinician lack of knowledge about non-binary genders. For non-binary young people who seek to access services and who receive poorly informed or pathologising responses, this is most certainly likely to contribute to poor outcomes. As such, a concerted focus on non-binary young people into the future in the clinical literature will be important, including consideration of how the GENDER mnemonic may or may not be applicable to non-binary young people. Whilst cisgenderism is a shared experience across non-binary young people and transgender young people who have a binary gender, its impacts are likely to be different.

Another area that requires ongoing attention are the effects of trauma upon transgender young people. Saketopoulou (2014), writing from the perspective of psychoanalysis, emphasises two forms that trauma may take, both of which are shaped by cisgenderism, namely being misgendered, and experiences of dysphoria. As Saketopoulou notes, neither are inherent to transgender young people (absent of cisgenderism), and neither are constitutive of pathology *per se*. Rather, Saketopoulou makes the point that both can lead to poor outcomes if transgender young people are not supported to address them. As Saketopoulou notes, in some ways this is a bit of a chicken and egg argument: if transgender young people are not the cause of misgendering or dysphoria, then why must they work on them? Yet as Saketopoulou notes, trauma arising from external forces is nonetheless trauma: it is not the product of the person who experiences it, but it will be detrimental to them *not* to address it. Certainly with some of the young people I work with, trauma is a significant part of our work. This may be due to experiences of cisgenderism with family or at school. It may be about the effects of dysphoria that have been minimised by the young person or their parents in a rush to be affirming. And for some young people it can be a product of the overwhelmingness of living in a society that is so marginalising of transgender young people.

This point about trauma brings me back to what I see as the difference between affirming approaches and an approach that takes a critical developmental approach to being affirming. As Saketopoulou (2014) suggests, affirming young people as experts on their gender, and doing so by challenging the equation of assigned sex with gender, potentially does very little to actually engage with cisgenderism. Indeed, as Saketopoulou suggests, the types of 'wrong body' narratives that are so prevalent in public narratives about transgender people's lives are in many ways reinforced when transgender young people's feelings of dysphoria are minimised. It is not reasonable to expect young people to exist outside of dominant narratives about embodiment. It is not reasonable to expect young people to parse their own embodiment outside of cisgenderist narratives that frequently tell young people their bodies are 'wrong'. Importantly, my point here is not to suggest that transgender young people should dislike their bodies, nor is it to reify one particular type of transgender body (i.e., the body that has never been through puberty associated with assigned sex, or the body that has 'completed' gender transition). This would constitute yet another form of transnormativity (Vipond 2015). Rather, it is to suggest that *speaking* about bodies is vitally important. Pretending bodies, in whatever form they take, don't exist so as to minimise dysphoria may ultimately be counterproductive.

Needed, then, is ongoing attention to how as clinicians we speak about bodies with transgender young people in ways that are not triggering in terms of dysphoria, but which nonetheless do not avoid the topic of embodiment. For many young people I work with there is a period of time where we tend not to talk about embodiment (and I refrain from specifically asking about it unless a young person raises the topic). This is about establishing trust and an attachment relationship where difficult topics can be broached. But over time I find we are able to talk about bodies, about the joys of having a body – a body that 'does what it needs to do' – but also the challenges that some (though certainly not all) young people experience in relation to their body. To me this is critical developmental work: it is about seeing the specificities of young transgender people's experiences, acknowledging that young people are often more than capable of doing the work to address trauma, and doing the work with them. For me, Saketopoulou (2014) encapsulates in the following sentence the kernel of the work I do in this regard: "the body one has needs to be known to the patient *so that, when necessary, it may eventually be given up*" (p. 782, emphasis in original). When it comes to hormone therapies and gender affirming surgeries in particular, for the young people I work with who want these, not having come to know *the body they have* is, in my experience, indicative of poor outcomes. Chaplin (2016) acknowledges this in her research with transgender adults who have had gender affirming surgeries. For those who were disengaged from their bodies, bodily changes following surgery were often configured as unknowable, given there had been no acknowledgement of the body before surgery. Certainly I recognise that engaging with the body you have when it isn't the body you want is difficult. It is traumatic. But my suggestion here is that it isn't a trauma we can productively shy away from.

Working with trauma, then, is necessarily complex. Yet to date much of the research on transgender young people and trauma has been focused on traumas purposively caused by others (i.e., by family members or abusive partners or strangers). Yet there are other traumas that are less commonly examined. These are still externally imposed (i.e., due to cisgenderism), but that they come to be part of the person's sense of themselves as transgender, as Saketopoulou (2014) argues, is why they too need concerted attention. To have a positive sense of oneself as transgender, in the face of cisgenderism, requires having carefully examined what it means to be transgender, including with regards to one's embodiment. This, of course, is part and parcel of the work that many transgender people do in coming to a place of self-knowing. My argument here is that suitably informed and skilled clinicians have an important role to play in facilitating this work.

A final area that requires ongoing attention pertains to transgender young people who are diagnosed with Autism Spectrum Disorder (ASD). Some researchers have suggested that there might be slightly elevated rates of ASD amongst transgender young people, though other research has contradicted this finding (May et al. 2017). A recent attempt by researchers (Strang et al. 2018) to use expert consensus to develop guidelines for the treatment of transgender young people who are diagnosed with ASD failed to gain consensus on key assumptions that are often made about such young people, namely that (1) an over focus on gender amongst young people 'causes' them to be transgender, (2) young people might 'confuse' sexuality with gender, and (3) ASD can lead to poor treatment compliance for transgender young people. The lack of expert consensus with regards to these particular assumptions is notable, given that such assumptions are often used to justify denying that a young person is transgender if they have received an ASD diagnosis.

Still, clinicians often seek to understand if there is a relationship between ASD and being transgender. Kennedy (2013) suggests that any relationship may be a product of some children diagnosed with ASD being less attuned to cisgenderism, and hence more willing to disclose that they are transgender. Jack (2012) suggests differently, proposing that transgender people may be especially attuned to normative gender ideologies, and may seek to proliferate or multiply gender categories so as to identify categories that better represent their gender. Jack also suggests that transgender young people diagnosed with ASD may focus less on the types of assumptions about what determines gender as outlined in Chap. 2, and instead may focus on specific details that signal to them something about gender. However we might seek to understand the relationship between ASD and being transgender, what is important is that clinicians do not conflate the two, or attempt to explain one away through recourse to the other, given this can lead to clinicians not affirming a young person's gender, or failing to address concerns related to being on the spectrum (Riggs and Bartholomaeus 2017).

Concluding Thoughts

Addressing trauma that is a product of cisgenderism, in whatever form, whether it be interpersonal violence or the impact of social norms upon a person's sense of self, will always be an ongoing task. As such, clinicians must face up to the difficult work of dismantling cisgenderism. Like any form of marginalisation, like any ideology, it will be resistant to change. It will permutate. The pathologising clinician who adopts a 'curative' approach may be slowly going the way of the dodo, but this does not mean that new forms of cisgenderism won't take its place and that subtler forms of cisgenderism don't already exist. Whether this be through the use of cisgenderist language, the gatekeeping of services, or the injunction that transgender people experience to explain themselves in order to access services, cisgenderism is never one singular thing that can be done away with. Nonetheless, it must be challenged. Clinicians need to be constantly attuned to its iterations, willing to stand up and be counted in terms of resisting normative gender ideologies.

Resistance can mean educating: educating each other, parents, schools, the media, and other institutions. It can mean challenging accepted 'best practice', including by establishing new practice guidelines and protocols based on community views (and making sure these are actually implemented); re-evaluating what is included in training curricula; conducting research in partnership with transgender communities; and speaking out against false claims made about transgender people's lives (such as 'rapid onset gender dysphoria') and those who would endorse them (which includes a particular cohort of clinicians, see Ansara and Hegarty 2012). It is about working collaboratively with transgender young people, but also about being accountable for one's role as a clinician in a system with long histories of cisgenderism and contemporary practices of gatekeeping. The 'good' cisgender clinician (given cisgender clinicians constitute the majority of clinicians who work with transgender young people) is not the 'perfect' clinician. Rather, the good cisgender clinician is one who acknowledges that they are part of a system that has often done harm, and that this requires accountability.

Whether it be helping a young person amend their birth certificate or make a legal name change, engaging with parents so that they are able to affirm a child, or speaking out publicly about the differential needs of transgender young people, these are all the role of the critical clinician who adopts an affirming approach. It is a role that eschews developmentalism, but nonetheless understands how gender is shaped across people's lives in response to cisgenderism. Cisgenderism cannot be all that we address in our work – there are joys as well as challenges – but a consideration of challenges must continue to be, at least for the foreseeable future, part of our core business.

References

Ansara, Y. G., & Hegarty, P. (2012). Cisgenderism in psychology: Pathologising and misgendering children from 1999 to 2008. *Psychology & Sexuality, 3*(2), 137–160.
Bartholomaeus, C., & Riggs, D. W. (2017). *Transgender people and education.* New York: Palgrave Macmillan.
Braun, V. (2000). Heterosexism in focus group research: Collusion and challenge. *Feminism & Psychology, 10*(1), 133–140.
Brown, S., Kucharska, J., & Marczak, M. (2018). Mental health practitioners' attitudes towards transgender people: A systematic review of the literature. *International Journal of Transgenderism, 19*(1), 4–24.
Chaplin, B. (2016). *"Why are you crying? You got what you wanted!": Psychosocial experiences of sex reassignment surgery.* Unpublished PhD thesis, Queensland University of Technology.
Clark, B. A., Veale, J. F., Townsend, M., Frohard-Dourlent, H., & Saewyc, E. (2018). Non-binary youth: Access to gender-affirming primary health care. *International Journal of Transgenderism, 19*(2), 158–169.
Gridley, S. J., Crouch, J. M., Evans, Y., Eng, W., Antoon, E., Lyapustina, M., et al. (2016). Youth and caregiver perspectives on barriers to gender-affirming health care for transgender youth. *Journal of Adolescent Health, 59*(3), 254–261.
Jack, J. (2012). Gender copia: Feminist rhetorical perspectives on an autistic concept of sex/gender. *Women's Studies in Communication, 35*(1), 1–17.
Kennedy, N. (2013). Cultural cisgenderism: Consequences of the imperceptible. *Psychology of Women Section Review, 15*(2), 3–11.
May, T., Pang, K., & Williams, K. J. (2017). Gender variance in children and adolescents with autism spectrum disorder from the National Database for Autism Research. *International Journal of Transgenderism, 18*(1), 7–15.
Meadow, T. (2018). *Trans kids: Being gendered in the twenty-first century.* Oakland: University of California Press.
Pullen Sansfaçon, A., Robichaud, M. J., & Dumais-Michaud, A. A. (2015). The experience of parents who support their children's gender variance. *Journal of LGBT Youth, 12*(1), 39–63.
Pullen Sansfaçon, A. P., Hébert, W., Lee, E. O. J., Faddoul, M., Tourki, D., & Bellot, C. (2018). Digging beneath the surface: Results from stage one of a qualitative analysis of factors influencing the well-being of trans youth in Quebec. *International Journal of Transgenderism, 19*(2), 184–202.

Riggs, D. W. (2019). An examination of 'just in case' arguments as they are applied to fertility preservation for transgender people. In V. Mackie, S. Ferber, & N. Marks (Eds.), *The body and the globe: From IVF to global reproductive industry*. New York: Lexington Books.

Riggs, D. W., & Bartholomaeus, C. (2015). The role of school counsellors and psychologists in supporting transgender people. *The Australian Educational and Developmental Psychologist, 32*(2), 158–170.

Riggs, D. W., & Bartholomaeus, C. (2016). Australian mental health professionals' competencies for working with trans clients: A comparative study. *Psychology & Sexuality, 7*(3), 225–238.

Riggs, D. W., & Bartholomaeus, C. (2017). The disability and diagnosis nexus: Transgender men navigating mental health care services. In C. Loeser, V. Crowley, & B. Pini (Eds.), *Disability and masculinities: Corporeality, pedagogy, and the critique of otherness* (pp. 67–84). London: Palgrave.

Riggs, D. W., & Bartholomaeus, C. (2018a). Fertility preservation decision making amongst Australian transgender and non-binary adults. *Reproductive Health, 15*, 181–191.

Riggs, D. W., & Bartholomaeus, C. (2018b). Gaslighting in the context of clinical interactions with parents of transgender children. *Sexual and Relationship Therapy, 33*, 382–394.

Riggs, D. W., & Sion, R. (2017). Gender differences in cisgender psychologists' and trainees' attitudes toward transgender people. *Psychology of Men & Masculinity, 18*(2), 187.

Saketopoulou, A. (2014). Mourning the body as bedrock: Developmental considerations in treating transsexual patients analytically. *Journal of the American Psychoanalytic Association, 62*(5), 773–806.

Smith, E., Jones, T., Ward, R., Dixon, J., Mitchell, A., & Hillier, L. (2014). *From blues to rainbows: The mental health and well-being of gender diverse and transgender young people in Australia*. Melbourne: Australian Research Centre in Sex, Health and Society (ARCSHS), La Trobe University.

Strang, J. F., Meagher, H., Kenworthy, L., de Vries, A. L., Menvielle, E., Leibowitz, S., & Pleak, R. R. (2018). Initial clinical guidelines for co-occurring autism spectrum disorder and gender dysphoria or incongruence in adolescents. *Journal of Clinical Child & Adolescent Psychology, 47*(1), 105–115.

Telfer, M., Tollit, M., Pace, C., & Pang, K. (2017). *Australian standards of care and treatment guidelines: For trans and gender diverse children and adolescents*. Melbourne: The Royal Children's Hospital.

Thorne, N., Witcomb, G. L., Nieder, T., Nixon, E., Yip, A., & Arcelus, J. (2018, Online First). A comparison of mental health symptomatology and levels of social support in young treatment seeking transgender individuals who identify as binary and non-binary. *International Journal of Transgenderism*, 1–10. https://doi.org/10.1080/15532739.2018.1452660.

Vipond, E. (2015). Resisting transnormativity: Challenging the medicalization and regulation of trans bodies. *Theory in Action, 8*(2), 21–44.

World Professional Association for Transgender Health (WPATH). (2011). *Standards of care for the health of transsexual, transgender, and gender nonconforming people, 7th version.*

Author Index

A

Ansara, Y. Gavriel, xiii, 6, 14, 140
Aramburu Alegría, Christine, 90

B

Bem, Sandra L., 40, 44, 45
Berenbaum, Sheri A., 35, 84, 107, 108

C

Castañeda, Claudia, 50–52

E

Ehrensaft, Diane, 14, 15, 18, 24, 109, 110, 113, 114

F

Fausto-Sterling, Anne, 33, 34, 36

J

John, Ian D., 3, 4, 7–10, 12, 27

K

Krieger, Irwin, 15

L

Lev, Arlene Istar, 11, 12, 18
Liben, Lynn S., 35, 84, 107, 108

M

Mallon, Gerald P., 12

Malpas, Jean, 13
McGuire, Jenifer K., 66
Meadow, Tey, 90, 92, 94, 118, 132
Menvielle, Edgardo, 12, 13
Morrow, Virginia, 115–117

Nealy, Elijah C., 16
Norwood, Kristen, 89, 94

Owen Blakemore, Judith E., 35, 84, 107, 108, 113

Pyne, Jake, 52, 97–99

Rahilly, Elizabeth P., 86, 95
Riggs, Damien W., 6, 17, 79, 83, 86, 94, 116, 127, 128, 132, 133, 135, 139
Ryan, Krysti N., 87, 92, 98, 99

Singh, Anneliese A., 52, 74

Tando, Darlene, 13, 14, 22, 110
Tilsen, Julie, 14

Wren, Bernadette, 88, 91

Subject Index

A

Advocacy, 21, 24, 61, 71, 74, 75, 79
American Psychiatric Association, 46, 47, 88
Animal companions, 105–120

B

Body, 6, 7, 15, 47, 60, 64–68, 79, 80, 96, 126, 135, 137, 138
Brother, *see* Siblings
Bullying, 20, 69, 119
 See also Discrimination; Harassment

C

Cisgenderism, vii–ix, xi, 6–9, 11–18, 22, 24–26, 32, 34, 39, 40, 42, 44–53, 58, 62, 64, 67, 72, 77, 80, 81, 83–102, 106, 107, 109, 112–118, 120, 124–131, 133, 135–140
Clinicians, ix–xii, 1–4, 7–13, 15, 16, 18–27, 32, 38, 45, 53, 58, 59, 64, 69, 73–76, 80, 81, 85, 91, 92, 98, 101, 114, 120, 124–140
Clothing, 42, 86–88, 92
Critical developmental approach, viii, 2, 21, 27, 32, 123, 124, 137

D

Developmentalism, viii, 12, 14, 17, 27, 32, 45–53, 98, 123, 133, 140

Developmental literature, 25, 58, 84, 86, 101, 106, 107
Diagnosis, ix, 11, 17, 18, 21, 45–48, 50, 64, 65, 88, 98, 130, 139
  See also Diagnostic and Statistical Manual of Mental Disorders (DSM); Diagnostic tools
Diagnostic and Statistical Manual of Mental Disorders (DSM), 46–50
Diagnostic tools, 32, 45, 46, 88
  See also Diagnosis; *Diagnostic and Statistical Manual of Mental Disorders* (DSM)
Disclose, *see* Disclosure
Disclosure, 48, 61, 64, 84, 87, 110, 113, 119
Discrimination, 2, 11, 13, 15, 16, 18, 20, 62, 64–69, 76, 109, 115, 116, 129
  See also Bullying; Harassment
Distress, 20, 22, 23, 39, 43, 47, 49, 50, 52, 57, 58, 60–71, 80, 83, 88, 92, 96, 106, 107, 114, 115, 118, 119, 131, 133
  See also GENDER mnemonic, distress management
DSM, *see Diagnostic and Statistical Manual of Mental Disorders*
DSM5, *see Diagnostic and Statistical Manual of Mental Disorders*
Dysphoria, *see* Gender dysphoria

Father, *see* Parents
Fertility, 25
  See also Fertility preservation
Fertility preservation, 21, 24, 133, 134
  See also Fertility

Gaslighting, 86, 135
Gender binaries, 8, 59, 60, 90, 128, 130
Gender categories, 6, 33, 37, 42, 139
Gender development
  gender intensification, 59–64, 66, 67, 75, 77
  gender schema theory, 44–45
  social learning approach, 40–41
  socio-cognitive approach, 41–44
Gender dysphoria, 47–49, 64, 80, 88, 132, 133, 140
Gender expression and parents
  channelling, 86–88
  differential treatment, 89–91
  direct instruction, 91–93
  modelling, 93–96
GENDER mnemonic
  distress management, 22
  ecologies of support, 23, 26, 117, 123
  expressed concerns, 20–21, 123
  gender journey and understanding, 19–20
  necessary actions, 21–22
  reinforcement and resistance, 23–24
Gender norms, 14, 18, 20, 61, 77, 78, 98
Gender presentation, 18, 90
Genitalia, 34–38, 42–45, 47, 53, 79, 80, 92, 95, 97
Grandparents, 26, 105–120

Harassment, 68
  See also Bullying; Discrimination

Subject Index   149

Hormones, 15, 20, 22, 52, 57, 59, 61, 63, 65–67, 70, 80, 133, 135, 138
See also Puberty blockers

Intimacy, 25, 70, 71, 75, 76, 78–80
See also Sexuality

Language, 7, 15, 33–38, 40, 73, 79, 80, 84, 131, 140
See also Pronouns
Loss, 17, 21, 26, 83, 89–91, 93, 95, 96, 99, 100, 114, 120, 124

Mental health, xi, 3, 7, 9, 15, 17, 32, 69, 72, 97, 105, 126–128, 134, 135
Misgender, 7, 23, 36, 66, 68, 69, 109, 111, 125, 128, 136
Mother, see Parents

Non-binary, 23–25, 95, 126, 129, 130, 135, 136

Online, 50, 71, 73–75, 79

Parents, x–xii, 11, 13–26, 31–33, 35–39, 43, 44, 50–54, 60–62, 65, 68–70, 72–75, 79, 83–102, 105, 106, 110–114, 118–120, 124–128, 132, 133, 135, 136, 140
Pathologising, 10, 25, 46, 50, 93, 96, 102, 105, 126, 136, 139
Play, 2, 10, 17, 23, 34, 35, 37–40, 46, 53, 61, 64, 73, 74, 79, 80, 86, 94, 96, 97, 107, 108, 113, 116, 120, 132, 138
Pronouns, 7, 34–37, 43, 68, 69, 87, 110, 111, 113
Puberty, 20, 25, 52, 57–80, 126, 133, 137
See also Puberty blockers
Puberty blockers, 22, 52, 57, 58, 61, 63, 65, 68–70, 72, 133, 135
See also Hormones

School, 17, 20, 21, 43, 44, 49–53, 61, 64, 68, 69, 72, 87, 88, 92, 106, 111, 132
Scientist-practitioner, 1–11, 26, 27, 32, 54, 127, 131
Sex differences, 4, 5
Sexuality, 78, 79, 93, 139
See also Intimacy
Siblings, 17, 26, 35, 43, 105–120
Sister, see Siblings
Standards of Care (SOC), 50–52, 126

World Professional Association for Transgender Health (WPATH), 50, 126

GPSR Compliance
The European Union's (EU) General Product Safety Regulation (GPSR) is a set of rules that requires consumer products to be safe and our obligations to ensure this.

If you have any concerns about our products, you can contact us on

ProductSafety@springernature.com

In case Publisher is established outside the EU, the EU authorized representative is:

Springer Nature Customer Service Center GmbH
Europaplatz 3
69115 Heidelberg, Germany

www.ingramcontent.com/pod-product-compliance
Ingram Content Group UK Ltd.
Pitfield, Milton Keynes, MK11 3LW, UK
UKHW021324180426

11947UKWH00017B/1421

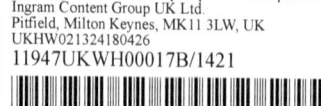